FOUR WAYS TO
CLICK

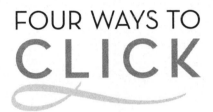

FOUR WAYS TO
CLICK

Rewire Your Brain for Stronger,
More Rewarding Relationships

Amy Banks, M.D.,

with Leigh Ann Hirschman

JEREMY P. TARCHER/PENGUIN | A MEMBER OF PENGUIN GROUP (USA) | NEW YORK

JEREMY P. TARCHER/PENGUIN
Published by the Penguin Group
Penguin Group (USA) LLC
375 Hudson Street
New York, New York 10014

USA · Canada · UK · Ireland · Australia
New Zealand · India · South Africa · China

penguin.com
A Penguin Random House Company

Most Tarcher/Penguin books are available at special quantity discounts for bulk
purchase for sales promotions, premiums, fund-raising, and educational needs.
Special books or book excerpts also can be created to fit specific needs. For details,
write: Special.Markets@us.penguingroup.com.

Library of Congress Cataloging-in-Publication Data

Banks, Amy Elizabeth.
Four ways to click : rewire your brain for stronger, more rewarding
relationships / Amy Banks, M.D., with Leigh Ann Hirschman.
p.   cm.
Includes bibliographical references and index.
ISBN 978-0-399-16919-9
1. Interpersonal relations.   2. Social psychology.   3. Brain.
I. Hirschman, Leigh Ann.   II. Title.
HM1106.B366   2015   2014035233
302—dc23

Printed in the United States of America
10   9   8   7   6   5   4   3   2   1

Book design by Ellen Cipriano

To

Jayme and Alex

for the love and joy that

fuel my life

CONTENTS

FOREWORD

Want to have more joy and contentment in your life? All the scientific studies of happiness, longevity, and mental and medical health point to one factor: the strength of your relationships with others. In *Four Ways to Click*, psychiatrist Amy Banks, M.D., provides an innovative and user-friendly summary of the extensive research on the neuroscience of relationships and offers readers practical ways to use this knowledge to retrain their brains for healthier, more rewarding relationships. What's in this for you? Simply put, you can intentionally transform your life by improving how you connect with others. Relationships are not simply the "icing on the cake" for a life well lived. *Relationships are the cake.*

After decades of studying how culture shapes our relationships as well as working as a psychiatrist in clinical practice, Amy Banks has brilliantly created what she calls the C.A.R.E. system, which can help improve the four ways we "click" with one another: how *calm* we feel around others, are *accepted* by others, *resonate* with the inner states of others, and are *energized* by these connections. Using the C.A.R.E. system as it is described in this book, readers can target the neural pathways that need fine-tuning so that the quality of their relationships increases. With an understanding of how our brains truly work we can intentionally change how we live our lives!

I love this book! It is beautifully written, engaging, and inspiring.

Want more happiness? Want to live longer? Want to be healthier in mind and body? Then learning these four ways to click into more meaningful and rewarding relationships is your passport to achieving these goals. Let Amy Banks be your guide to a better life of love and laughter. Enjoy!

—DANIEL J. SIEGEL, M.D.

Chapter 1

BOUNDARIES ARE OVERRATED

A New Way of Looking at Relationships

Boundaries are overrated.

If you want healthier, more mature relationships; if you want to stop repeating old patterns that cause you pain; if you are tired of feeling emotionally disconnected from the people you spend your time with; if you want to grow your inner life, you can begin by questioning the idea that there is a clear, crisp line between you and the people you interact with most frequently.

People who talk a lot about boundaries tend to make statements like these:

"It shouldn't matter what other people do and say to you, not if you have a strong sense of self."

"How do parents know they've been successful? When their children no longer need them."

"Best friends and true romance are for the young. As you get older, you naturally grow apart from other people."

"You shouldn't need other people to complete you."

"You wouldn't have so many problems if you would just stand on your own two feet."

The message is clear: it's not "healthy" to need other people—and whatever you do, don't let yourself be infected by other peoples' feelings, thoughts, and emotions. The statements above are intended to have an emotional effect on you. You may notice that they sound just a *teensy* bit judgmental and shaming. I know they make me uncomfortable; when I read them, I feel like I'm standing in a harsh white spotlight with someone pointing a finger at me, intoning *You're pretty messed up, missy, and it's all your fault.*

The ideal of complete psychological independence is one that was very big with mental health professionals in much of the twentieth century, and it still has our culture by the throat. So even if those statements about boundaries carry a sting, they also probably sound familiar to you, or even self-evident. Obvious!

So I couldn't possibly be suggesting that they're untrue. I couldn't possibly say that it can be good to be dependent, or that our mental health is unavoidably affected by the people we share our lives with, or that we achieve emotional growth when we are profoundly connected to others instead of when we are apart from them.

That's exactly what I'm saying.

This book is going to show you a different way of thinking about your emotional needs and what it means to be a healthy, mature adult. A new field of scientific study, one I call *relational neuroscience,* has shown us that there is hardwiring throughout our brains and bodies designed to help us engage in satisfying emotional connection with others. This hardwiring includes four primary neural pathways that are featured in this book. Relational neuroscience has also shown that when we are cut off from others, these neural pathways suffer. The result is a neurological cascade that can result in chronic irritability and anger, depression, addiction, and chronic physical illness. We are just not as healthy when we try to stand on our own, and that's because the human brain is built to operate within a network of caring human relationships. How do we reach our personal and professional potential? By being warmly, safely connected to partners, friends, coworkers, and family. Only then do our neural pathways get the stimulation they need to make our brains calmer, more tolerant, more resonant, and more productive.

The good news for those of us whose relationships don't always feel so warm or safe: it is possible to heal and strengthen those four neural pathways that are weakened when you don't have strong connections. Relationships and your brain form a virtuous circle, so by strengthening your neural pathways for connection, you will also make it easier to build the healthy relationships that are essential for your psychological and physical health.

For many people, the news about the importance of relationships began with a 1998 study at the University of Parma in Italy, a study that proved how deeply connected we are to one another, right down to our neurons.

Your Feelings, My Brain

It was one of those lucky scientific mistakes, an unexpected observation that could have easily gone unnoticed if it hadn't been for an astute researcher. When Giacomo Rizzolatti, a neurophysicist at the University of Parma, and his research team began their now-famous experiment, they were not intending to explore how human beings interact. In fact, they were not even studying people. The Italian researchers were mapping a small area, known as *F5*, in the brains of the macaque monkey. At this point in neurological research, it was already well known that the F5 neurons fire when a monkey reaches his arm and hand away from his body to grasp an object.

One routine day in the lab, a researcher observed something unprecedented. The researcher was standing in the line of sight of a monkey whose F5 cells had been implanted with micro-sized electrodes. As the researcher reached out to grasp an object, the electrodes placed on the monkey's F5 area activated.

Remember: it was known that the F5 neurons activate when a monkey moves his arm to grasp something.

Then think about this: the monkey was not moving *his* arm; he was simply watching as the *researcher's* arm moved.

This seemed impossible. At the time of this observation, scientists believed that the nerve cells for action were separate and distinct from the nerve cells for sensory observations. Sensory neurons picked up information from the outside world; motor neurons were devoted to acting. So when the F5 area, known for its link to physical action, lit up in the brain of a monkey who was only *watching* action in someone else, it was a clear violation of this known divide. It was as if the brain of the monkey and the brain of the researcher were somehow synchronized. Even more unsettling, it was as if their brains overlapped, as if the researcher's physical movement existed inside the monkey.[1]

As Rizzolatti and other neuroscientists pursued this odd observation, they found that human brains also demonstrate this mirroring effect. In other words, you understand me by performing an act of internal mimicry—by letting some of my actions and feelings into your head. Ask a friend to briskly rub her hands together as you watch. Chances are that as her hands become warm from the friction, your hands will start to feel warm, too. In the aftermath of the monkey experiment, it was hypothesized that our brains contain mirror neurons, nerve cells that are dedicated to the task of imitating others. Most scientists no longer feel that specific mirror neurons exist; instead, there is a brainwide mirroring system whose tasks are shared by a number of regions and pathways. The imitating effect—the reason your hands warm up when your friend rubs hers together—happens because neural circuits throughout your brain are copying what you hear and see. Nerves in your frontal and prefrontal cortex (the same ones that are activated when you plan to rub your own hands together and then execute that plan) begin to fire. At the same time, neurons in your somatosensory cortex, which is the area of the brain responsible for bodily sensations, activate and send you messages of friction and warmth. Deep inside your brain, *your* hands are rubbing themselves together—even if your hands don't actually move.

Actually, the process goes far beyond the mere reflection of another person's actions. Your mirroring system is made up of neurons that can "see" or "hear" what someone else is doing. The system then recruits neurons from other areas of the brain to provide you with input not just about sensations and actions but about emotions, too. This input lets you have a comprehensive, detailed imitation of what the other person is experiencing. That's why you can almost instantly pick up on the emotion of another person. If you watch as I rub my hands together, your brain might read the excitement on my face as I demonstrate how the mirroring system works—and *you* may feel some of that excitement. If you've ever "caught" a smile that you spotted on the face of a complete stranger, or if the silent tension of your partner has caused your own heart to race, you've experienced the effects of the mirroring system. This emotional contagion is caused by a neural pathway that can, in effect, take in another person's feelings and replicate them squarely inside you.

When I ask groups of people to try the hand-rubbing experiment, there are usually two sets of reactions. Some people are amazed, as if they've just watched themselves pull a rabbit out of a hat. Their neurological connection with others feels like magic. But other people immediately say, "This is creepy!"

I get it. When you've been taught all your life that your mind is its own little castle, one that's surrounded by a thick, high wall that's designed to keep your thoughts and feelings in and everyone else's out, it can be unsettling to learn about the power of the mirroring system. And in fact, the discovery of our mirroring ability challenges some traditional assumptions about how our brains and bodies are wired. Vittorio Gallese, a neurophysiologist in the Parma lab, described the role of the mirroring system in human interactions this way: "The neural mechanism is involuntary, with it we don't have to think about what other people are doing or feeling, we simply know."[2] Marco Iacoboni, a professor of psychiatry at UCLA, takes it one step further in his book *Mirroring People*. He says that the mirroring system helps us in "understanding our existential condition and our involvement with others. [It shows] that we are not alone, but are biologically wired and evolutionarily designed to be deeply interconnected with one another."[3]

When you and I interact, an impression of the interaction is left on my nervous system. I literally carry my contact with you around inside me, as a neuronal imprint. The next time you hear someone say, "Don't let other people affect how you feel," remember the mirroring system. Because we don't really have a choice. For good or for bad, other people affect us, and we are not as separate from one another as psychologists once thought.

Maturity Has a New Meaning

When I say that boundaries are overrated, I don't mean that there are absolutely no boundaries, or that all of humanity is just one big, undifferentiated, brownish-beige lump. Nor am I suggesting that anyone give up her or his own distinct personality for the sake of fitting in with a cozy, companionable group. No therapist I know believes that it's healthy to abandon your beliefs, preferences, and quirks for the sake of a smoothly running—and bland—larger whole.

For decades, in fact, psychology moved in the other direction, in the belief that the only path to human growth was traveled via emotional separation. According to separation-individuation theory, which was most energetically advanced by Margaret Mahler in the 1970s, we all begin our work of separation in the first six or seven months of life, when we start to realize that our caregiver is a person distinct from ourselves. Separation-individuation theory holds that the rest of life is a variation on this discovery. In the *practicing* stage of human development, we supposedly practice separation by crawling or toddling away from our mothers and then returning to their arms. In the *object constancy* stage, we develop the capacity to hold an abstract image of Mom in our minds, meaning that we are secure enough to venture farther and farther away from her, thus developing our independence. As school-aged children, we become more aggressive in an attempt to move forward with our individual desires. In adolescence, we move further away from our parents by developing a sexual identity and pairing off with our peers. Adulthood? It's a constant process of refining our ability to stand on our own, soothe our own distress, and solve our own problems. With each stage, the boundary between the self and other people grows stronger, more solid. Separation-individuation theory has been written about in thousands of books and dissertations, but here's a micro-summary: in order to grow, we must step farther and farther away from others. The fully mature person may enjoy other people but doesn't really *need* them. He is defined by the firm boundaries between himself and other people, and within those boundaries he is a self-sufficient being.

Even before the mirroring system came on the scene, and before relational neuroscience began to turn up additional evidence for the biological basis of human connectedness, some in the field wondered whether the separation model had gone too far. In the 1970s, a forward-looking group of Boston mental health experts—psychiatrist Jean Baker Miller and psychologists Judith V. Jordan, Irene Stiver, and Janet Surrey—noticed that their patients weren't suffering from poor boundaries. They weren't suffering from a lack of personal independence from others. What they suffered from was a lack of healthy human connection. As Judith Jordan notes, "The Separate Self model has wrongly suggested that we are intrinsically motivated to build firmer boundaries, gain power over other people in order to establish safety, and compete with others for scarce resources. Mutuality helps us see that human beings thrive in relationships in which both people are growing and contributing to good connection."[4]

When you look at relationships this way, it's possible to take the stages of development according to separation-individuation theory and cast them in a warmer light. When an infant crawls away from her mother, she's not trying to separate from humanity. Instead, the baby is expanding her relational world; she's moving toward *more* connections, toward the big world and the people who populate that world, before scooting back to enjoy her relationship with her mother. A toddler who learns object constancy isn't building the ability to get away from Mom; by developing a mental image of her mother, she's able to carry Mom with her wherever she goes. She's learning a skill necessary for sustaining relationships over distance and time. As school-aged children interact with their peers and make mistakes, they learn how to manage relationships. Teenagers expand their relational worlds even further; they negotiate sexual relationships, and they have to learn how to become part of a group without succumbing to peer pressure. This reinterpretation of developmental growth has an overarching theme: human beings don't mature by separating. Instead, they grow toward a greater and greater relational complexity. This approach to

human development has a name: *relational-cultural theory,*
or RCT. As a young psychiatrist, I found that RCT was
more effective than any other theory, including separation-
individuation, in helping people heal and helping them grow.
I've spent twenty years applying RCT to the problems of my
patients and the disconnected world they—and we—live in.

Separation theory and RCT have a few ideas in common:
to be healthy, you have to know who you are; what your feelings and thoughts are; that other people have thoughts and
feelings, too; and you have to be able to differentiate yourself
within a relationship. But in separation theory, you're learning all this in order to eventually walk away. You can still
forge bonds and be part of a community if you want to, but
your role as an adult has to be earned by your ability to tough
things out on your own. This is a psychology that emphasizes
a defensive stance, because you're always defining and pro-
tecting your boundaries. You're wary of being invaded by
other people's emotions and problems. In fact, this is how
Freud saw the condition of being alive: "For the living organ-
ism protection against stimuli is almost a more important
task than reception of stimuli."[5] It's sad, isn't it? In separation
theory, there is always a wall between you and other people.

In RCT, there are no walls between people. Good relationships are the rich soil in which people grow and bloom.
A good relationship with your parents helps you feel safe
enough to approach other people and make a connection with
them. A good relationship with your peers helps you try out

who you are, practice your skills of empathy, and learn communication. As your skills for relationship grow, so does your desire for more relationship.

Relational-cultural theory doesn't imagine people as defined by boundaries; it sees relationships as more like a magician's linking rings. The rings are a set, but they are not stuck in a rigid configuration. They can move far apart and they can move closer together. And they can—this is the magic part—temporarily interconnect and overlap, just as they do when you watch someone rub his hands together and feel the warmth in your own. Or when you sometimes feel like you're in another person's skin, finishing their sentences or feeling their sadness. There's flexibility and movement in this definition of relationship. You come together, experiencing each other; and then you move away again so that you can absorb what you've learned. Relationships are a dynamic process of experiencing, learning, and integrating your knowledge so that you are able to see both yourself and the other person more deeply and more clearly.

Jean Baker Miller liked to talk about "growth-fostering relationships," a wonderfully descriptive term that suggests just the right idea: relationships aren't an end in themselves. Although a relationship can be a safe harbor, it is never just that. It also helps you grow. A good relationship helps you and the other person develop clarity about yourselves; promotes your self-worth; makes you more productive at your work; and it gives you an appetite for more relationships. In Baker Miller's language, a growth-fostering relationship brings more "zest" to everything you do. When you're in a growth-fostering relationship, you're not being belittled or silenced, and you're not hiding from the things that bother you. A growth-fostering relationship is the opposite of having to put up walls and fortify the battlements. Instead, you are constantly reaching out to others and stretching toward greater maturity.

So for years before the mirroring study, I was using Relational-Cultural Theory, or RCT, to help my patients. Instead of giving struggling young people the standard advice to "separate from your parents and stop depending on them for emotional support," we looked for ways they could stay connected to their families of origin while building their adult lives. Instead of telling people with explosive anger or chronic irresponsibility that they had to learn to self-regulate, we picked their relationships that felt the most durable—and worked on new emotional skills in an atmosphere that made it safer and easier to take risks. Sometimes I saw patients who were barely hanging on, whose relational worlds were limited to one or two abusive connections. In these cases, we worked together to find ways to detach from unhealthy relationships and—gently, slowly—grow relationships that held more potential for acceptance and warmth. From these starting points, we'd continue the work that would allow them to grow, expand, connect, heal, and move forward. I grew, too, refusing to maintain a cool distance in the therapy room. Whereas a separation-individuation therapist would see it as her job to help her patients stand on their own, I forged real relationships with my clients. I shared my own worries and feelings and expanded my emotional repertoire. Within the relationship, the patient grew—and so did I. That's how RCT works. As one client said, "Relational therapy differed from my previous therapy, which was about me as an individual with no real connection to the therapist. In relational therapy, we worked together. The therapist went out of her way to make an emotional bond with me. I saw and felt her concern and caring."

Healthy Relationships = Healthy Body

From a clinical perspective—my private laboratory—this approach was working. I wasn't alone, either; my colleagues at the Jean Baker Miller Training Institute at the Wellesley Centers for Women were doing the same thing, with similar good results. Patients who came to us as chronic "hard cases"—the kind who are transferred from therapist to therapist and never seem to improve—blossomed. They became more able to derive gratification from real give-and-take relationships. Stressed-out people became calmer; the rejected became more trusting; the abusive developed empathy; and people who had emotionally flatlined became more energetic.

On a case-by-case basis, we had enough proof for our approach to keep going. Every day we saw people developing through and toward relationships, instead of away from them.

But we also were bolstered by the stunning evidence about the health benefits of relationships. This evidence could fill an entire book—and in his book *Love and Survival: The Scientific Basis for the Healing Power of Intimacy,* the trailblazing cardiologist Dean Ornish does amass hundreds of pages of studies and thinking about the subject. Here are just a few of the highlights:

- Researchers in North Carolina measured the effect of social support on 331 men and women, sixty-five years of age and older. After controlling for known risk factors like age, sex, race, economic status, diet, physical health status, stressful life events, and cigarette smoking, the researchers found that those who perceived their social support to be impaired had a *340 percent* higher rate of premature death than those who felt their social support was good.[6]

- A Yale University study looked at the coronary angiographs of 119 men and 40 women. (A coronary angiograph shows whether and to what extent your coronary arteries are blocked.) The patients who reported more "feelings of being loved" had far fewer blockages than those who didn't. The patients who felt loved had fewer blockages even than the patients who had busy social circles but who didn't feel particularly nurtured or supported. These findings held true even after the researchers accounted for genetic predisposition to heart disease and environmental risk factors like age, hostility, smoking, diet, and exercise.[7]

- In a long-term study that began in the 1940s, male medical students at Johns Hopkins filled out a questionnaire that assessed how close they felt to their parents. There were 1,100 students who participated in the study, all of them healthy at the time they completed the questionnaire. In a remarkable feat of logistics, the students were tracked down fifty years later. The students who had developed cancer in the intervening years were less likely to have had close relationships with their parents than students who did not have cancer. Interestingly, a poor relationship between the male student and his father was the strongest predictor of cancer. Again, these findings were independent of other known risks for cancer.[8]

- In the 1950s, Harvard students (all healthy, all men) were interviewed about the warmth and closeness of their mothers and fathers. They were also asked to describe their parents. Thirty-five years later, when the students were middle-aged, 29 percent who had good parental relationships and described their parents in positive terms had developed illnesses. But

95 percent of students who had poor relationships with their parents and who described their mothers and fathers in negative terms had become sick.[9]

Let these studies sink in for a moment. Better cardiovascular health. Fewer cases of cancer. Better health in midlife. And 340 percent fewer premature deaths from all causes. Here was clear evidence that the perception of having healthy human connection is critical not just for emotional health but physical health as well. When I was a child, the government was worried about curious kids who were drinking household chemicals and accidentally poisoning themselves. To address the problem, they distributed acid-green stickers decorated with the face of Mr. Yuk, who displayed a theatrically sick expression. Parents placed these stickers on dangerous chemicals throughout the house to send a clear warning message to their children who were too young to read. I've often thought we need a similarly strong message for adults about the poison of disconnection. Why don't medical waiting rooms offer pamphlets marked with a skull and crossbones, with the words *Social isolation can kill you* in stark letters underneath? The evidence for the claim is certainly there. Maybe a clear message like that would temper our compulsive need to stand on our own two feet.

The C.A.R.E. Plan

At the time Jean Baker Miller and her colleagues at Wellesley were forming their theories about human development, there was no technology available to see what was happening in the brain when it was either isolated or connected. Like everyone else at the time, the group had to work from their external observations. But then, in the 1990s, technology made brain study more possible. With advanced scanning technologies that allowed scientists to see the brain functioning in real time, and with discoveries such as learning that the brain can grow new cells even in old age, new findings about brain activity and new fields of research emerged. By the year 2000, neuroscientists were eagerly studying the brain's activity within the context of relationships. What they've found since then has taken relational-cultural therapy's work and extended it. The new science is completely upending the old ideas about separation and individuation.

Relational neuroscience has been showing that people cannot reach their full potential unless they are in healthy connection with others. Take the mirroring system. It needs relational input to stay in shape. So you need to really "see" other people (in the emotional sense that you understand and honor their feelings) *and* be "seen" in order to keep the mirroring system functioning well; without that input, it's harder to perceive other people accurately and to feel close to them. There are other neural pathways, too, that are nurtured when we are in good relationships. Other systems use the input from healthy relationships to help tell our brains to turn off the stress response, to think clearly, and to feel pleasure without resorting to damaging or addictive behavior. (The next chapter describes the scientific findings in more detail.)

It's important to stay humbled by the knowledge of how much we still don't know about the brain and relationships. As always, we can only work with the best knowledge available. But the knowledge we *do* have has provided me with a way of talking to my patients about how relationships are vehicles for our growth and our healing. It helps people really "get" why relationships are so crucial to feeling happier, to managing their stress, to feeling less angry, to stop eating or shopping or drinking compulsively, or to make other changes. It's also provided the framework for a plan that blends relational psychology and neuroscience to help patients make those changes.

Remember when I said that good relationships help people feel calmer, more tolerant, more resonant, and more productive? Each of these four benefits of a healthy relationship is directly related to a specific neural pathway. These pathways help you feel:

Calm. A feeling of calm is regulated in part by a pathway of the autonomic nervous system called the *smart vagus.* When you're feeling stressed, your primitive brain wants to kick in—and when the primitive brain is in charge, it tends to make decisions that are bad news for relationships. When you have strong relationships, the smart vagus can modulate the stress response and keep the primitive brain from taking over. You're healthier, can think more clearly, and you're more likely to solve problems through creative thinking instead of exploding in anger or running away. But when you're isolated from other people, your smart vagus can suffer from what neuroscientists call *poor tone*. This means that your primitive brain is more likely to call the shots. In the short term, this leads to relationship problems. Over time, you can expect chronic stress, illness, depression, and big-time irritability.

Accepted. A sense of belonging flows from a well-functioning dorsal anterior cingulate cortex, or dACC. The role of the dorsal anterior cingulate cortex is featured in SPOT, or *social pain overlap theory*, in which scientists show that being left out hurts—physically. Unfortunately, a person who suffers frequent exclusion can develop a dorsal anterior cingulate cortex that is highly reactive to social pain, leaving him or her to sense rejection even when other people are welcoming. Have you ever known someone who snaps at you when you say something mild and friendly like, "Hey, you look a little tired today. Are you all right?" Then you know someone who may be suffering from an overactive dorsal anterior cingulate cortex.

Resonant. Resonance with other people—the feeling among friends who "get" each other—is facilitated by the mirroring system. As I've described, other people's experiences are imprinted onto our nervous system in a very literal way. When your mirroring pathways are weak, it's hard to read other people or even to send out signals that allow other people to accurately read *you*.

Energetic. Energy is a benefit of the relational brain's dopamine reward system. In the beginning—whenever that was—human beings were created with a clever, life-enhancing mechanism that exists to this day. When we're engaged in healthy, growth-promoting activities, we are rewarded with a hit of dopamine that sweeps through the body's reward circuitry, producing a wave of euphoria and energy. Dopamine's feel-good effects are the carrot on the stick for healthy behavior: water, healthy nutrition, sex, and human relationships all stimulate dopamine. It was such a simple and ingenious plan . . . until casinos, malls, and opium dens came along. Sigh. When people don't get enough pleasure from healthy relationships, they may turn to less healthy sources like addictive shopping, drugs, or compulsive sex to get their dopamine hits. And when they do this enough, they can rewire their brains so that the dopamine pathways are no longer connected to relationships. Even when they're in a good relationship, some people just can't get real enjoyment from it.

Calm. Accepted. Resonant. Energetic.

Each of these four pathways is a feedback loop. Supply the loop with good relationships, and most of the time, the pathway will become stronger. Strengthen the pathway, and your relationships become more rewarding. There are plenty of places in each loop to step in and boost the entire system.

This book describes what I call the C.A.R.E. program,

named after the four benefits of a healthy relationship. The C.A.R.E. program is the book version of work I've been doing with clients for fifteen years. It can help heal some of the neural damage that isolation or chronic emotional disconnection can cause. It can also help you form healthy, thriving connections—whether you need a new perspective on one particularly sticky relationship or whether you describe yourself as "just not good with people" and want a major relational overhaul. This program has also helped successfully address the symptoms that extend past the immediate pain of disconnection, including addictions, stress, anxiety, anger problems, and more.

In the first part of this book, I'll describe in detail the neuroscience of relationships, including the role of each of the four neural pathways. I'll also show you how the brain can make itself over, in ways that can be positive or negative. Depending on your emotional connections, your brain can either suffer the damage of rejection and isolation—or enjoy the healing benefits of growth-fostering relationships.

If a lack of healthy connection is a problem for you, at first the solution might seem to be simple: go out and make some friends. But of course it's *not* that simple, not in a society that underplays the importance of close relationships and overplays the need to be independent, judgmental, and separate. It is most certainly not simple if you have suffered neurological damage from chronic disconnection. In the second and very practical section of this book, the C.A.R.E. program will help you use psychological and relational neuroscience—together—to melt away unwanted neural pathways and create new ones that make it easier to forge healthy connections. You'll take a relationship inventory that reveals which of your neural pathways for connection are receiving good support, and which need shoring up. You'll also discover which of your relationships hold the most potential for growth. If you have relationships that are damaging your C.A.R.E. neural pathways and making it harder for you to connect, you'll learn that, too. These insights can help you heal the physical and emotional damage from disconnection and help you make relationships that really click.

With this information in hand, you can customize the C.A.R.E. program to your needs. The C.A.R.E. plan is laid out across four chapters, with one chapter for each of the neural pathways. You can work through the entire plan, or you can use the steps on an as-needed basis to target your neural pathways with specific treatments and exercises. Some of those treatments can be done alone; a few require a prescription or a specialist; and others you undertake within the context of your safest relationships. In general, though, the C.A.R.E. plan is a series of simple actions that strengthen your ability to connect at all levels, from the cellular to the behavioral. At the end of the program you will have relationships—some old ones and maybe some new ones—that feel calmer, safer, more zestful, and more mutual. It's time to start tearing down walls, and time to start healing your brain.

Chapter 2

THE FOUR NEURAL PATHWAYS
FOR HEALTHY RELATIONSHIPS

A culture telling you that you need to separate from others and be independent above all else is selling you an ancient script. Not one that's based on the brain as it is, but the brain as it *was*.

Years ago, when my children were young, they were given a kit for raising a frog from a tadpole. With much positive anticipation, we set up the frog habitat in the kitchen and ordered a tadpole we dubbed Uncle Milty. Uncle Milty's home was just beside the breakfast preparation area. Each morning, as I made breakfast for my kids, we would peek into the small container of water to see if Uncle Milty had sprouted his frog legs yet. Weeks went by. Milty's head and torso grew bigger and bigger, but . . . no legs. In our household, we talk a lot about the importance of relationships for good health and development, so it was natural for everyone to speculate: was it possible that Milty was not becoming a frog because he was alone in his habitat? Like human babies who fail to thrive because they are not held, was Milty failing to grow legs because he didn't have another amphibian to cuddle with? Without relationships, would he remain an immature, unsatisfied tadpole? No. Our family was trying to analyze Milty as if he had a human brain. But he didn't. He had a reptile brain.

Reptiles and amphibians have brains that, basically, haven't evolved in about five hundred million years. The reptile brain doesn't need relationships. It doesn't require connection with others for physical development. The reptile brain is all about bare-knuckled survival, about breathing, eating, reproducing, fighting, and hotfooting it away from anything that might want to eat it. Uncle Milty never did develop legs (the poor guy couldn't hotfoot away from anything), but he was probably the victim of a genetic mutation, not loneliness—because the reptile brain doesn't get lonely. It doesn't care about anyone else. It doesn't need anyone else. It's the very model of separation and rugged independence.

We humans still possess the primitive reptile brain; it's what we call our *brain stem*. But the brain stem is just one structure within a human brain that has evolved far beyond the reptile brain to be much larger, more complicated, and more advanced. The human brain is different from the reptile brain in a zillion ways, but the one I'm most concerned with here is that, over millennia, the human brain has evolved away from reptilian independence. For example, reptiles don't have neural equipment that causes them to feel pain if they are left out of a social group . . . but you and I do. Reptiles don't possess a nerve that uses signals from welcoming facial expressions to modulate stress . . . but you and I do. Reptiles don't need to know that other reptiles really "get" them . . . but we do. Reptiles don't get a surge of a motivating neurochemicals when they're in the company of others. . . . but . . . you get the picture.

Uncle Milty didn't need or want friends to be a fully developed frog, but our brains are different. To us, healthy connection is central. The old reptile script of surviving on your own, of not needing others to help you develop and grow, is life threatening to mammals. It is life threatening to you. Fortunately, it is possible to write a new script, one that's more in tune with the reality of our human brains. Humans have developed a deep need to connect with others, and we're constantly learning more about the neurobiology that underpins our need for good relationships. This chapter will describe some of that neurobiology.

No single area of the brain exclusively regulates relationships; this is a function that appears to be integrated across many parts of the human nervous system. Although there's always a danger of oversimplification when it comes to describing neurobiology, I find it helpful to think about our human brain's need for connection in terms of the four major neural C.A.R.E. pathways I described in the last chapter. When you are in healthy relationships with others, your brain sends messages that help you feel:

Calm (this pathway is governed by the smart vagus
   nerve)
Accepted (ruled by the dorsal anterior cingulate
   cortex, or dACC)
Resonant (the mirroring system)
Energetic (the dopamine reward system)

The health and strength of these pathways are influenced
by early childhood relationships, and then these pathways are
reshaped continually throughout our lives, again in the context of our relationships. That's right: our relationships sculpt
our brains. The quality of our relationships helps determine
our ability to feel motivated, to remain coolheaded in a crisis,
and to perceive other people's social signals with accuracy.
This is exciting news; it means that even if our C.A.R.E. pathways aren't working very well, we can learn to leverage the
power of relationships to heal and change them. And we can
think differently about how we raise the next generation, so
that our children and grandchildren possess fully functioning
systems for connectedness.

C Is for Calm: The Smart Vagus

I'll begin with a story about Brooke, a client of mine. I'm bet-
ting that her story will sound familiar. Maybe you've lived it.
   After a stretch of unemployment, Brooke was delighted
to land a job just before the winter holidays. But she was

anguished, too, because her new employer was throwing her annual holiday party on the Friday of Brooke's first week of work. As the week progressed, Brooke was increasingly torn between the desire to make a good impression on her coworkers and her dread of socializing in a large, unfamiliar group. She imagined awkward conversations with colleagues she barely knew; the humiliating feeling of her sweaty hand in another's dry palm; the uncomfortable but liberating moment when a conversation partner declares that it is time to mingle with other people. Brooke resigned herself to an evening of stress and faking it for the sake of her career. Her only hope for escape was a sudden natural disaster or an open bar serving very large glasses of white wine.

The night of the party, Brooke entered the hotel lobby and immediately felt like an outsider. Everywhere she turned, small groups of people huddled together, talking. A few of the people seemed to be looking in her direction and smirking. *Get over yourself,* Brooke thought, *no one is laughing at you.* But she stood off to the side for nearly thirty minutes, sipping her wine and looking around in vain for a face that appeared even a little bit friendly.

Rescue arrived in the form of her coworker Pete, who greeted Brooke warmly and wished her happy holidays. Almost immediately, Brooke began to relax. She and Pete had met a few days earlier at an office lunch meeting. During a break in the meeting, she discovered they shared a similar sense of humor and an unusual hobby: fly-fishing. At the party, they picked up where they had left off at the meeting, swapping stories about streams that were off the beaten track and debating the best fly for catching a striped bass. The rest of the party went smoothly. Pete brought two of their colleagues into the discussion and Brooke introduced herself to a few more. Maybe it was the wine, Brooke remarked to herself, but the group seemed to become much friendlier and more open as the night went on.

It wasn't the wine. (Brooke had drunk very little.) Thanks to complex forces in Brooke's life, a pathway in her nervous system was unable to accurately read and respond to the people she saw when she entered the party. Instead of seeing welcoming faces, she saw mockery. Even when she tried to talk herself into seeing things differently (*Get over yourself, Brooke; no one is laughing at you*), she was nearly overpowered by a feeling of jeopardy, a feeling that no one wanted her around. But as she talked with her new friend Pete, that pathway in her nervous system, the smart vagus, started to do its job. Not only could Brooke relax, she was better able to transmit and receive social cues. She could show friendliness. She could *see* it on the faces of others.

The human central nervous system is the control center for the electrical activity that drives your thoughts and actions. It contains an essential subsystem: the *autonomic* (think automatic) *nervous system*, which is designed to help you quickly respond to threats or stress. The autonomic nervous system is at work 24/7, humming along below the level of your conscious awareness. It runs throughout your entire body, innervating muscles, organ systems, and glands. We used to think that our autonomic nervous system was a lot like Uncle Milty's, with only two major parts:

> The *sympathetic nervous system*, which is responsible
> for the famous fight-or-flight response.
> The *parasympathetic nervous system*, which leads to the
> freeze response.

In other words, scientists believed that when you feel surprised or threatened, your body automatically responds in one of two ways: either your sympathetic nervous system revs up, providing you with the energy and focus needed to fight or flee; or your parasympathetic nervous system activates, slowing your body processes down so that you freeze and play dead. According to most introductory biology and psychology courses, whether you fight, flee, or freeze is largely dependent on the extent of the threat and on your ability to man up to it. If the threat seems potentially survivable and you are large and strong, you face the threat head-on. If you face that same threat but are small and weak, it is better to turn and run as fast as you can. Those are the choices in the sympathetic nervous system's fight-or-flight response. In the face of a severe, life-threatening situation, you might do what the baby rabbit I found on my porch last spring did. The bunny, which had been dropped there by one of my cats as a special "gift" to me, looked dead. But it was actually in the midst of a full-blown freeze response, in which the parasympathetic nervous system exerts a slowing down or calming effect. The body and brain begin to shut down; they literally go numb. Ideally, this reaction causes the predator to lose interest and turn away, but if the predator keeps attacking, the freeze response creates protection from the tremendous pain and stress. This is where the expression "playing dead" comes from, but the freeze reaction is anything but play and is not under conscious control. This shutting down of bodily functions is so effective that one-quarter of the animals playing dead actually die. (Fortunately, when I separated the bunny from its predators for a few hours, the parasympathetic stimulation stopped and the bunny hopped away.) Obviously, this potentially lethal response is the last line of defense for any animal, including humans.

These reactions of the sympathetic and parasympathetic nervous systems, collectively named the "fight, flight, or freeze" responses, have been socially and scientifically accepted as the truth of how human beings respond to stress since they were identified by physiologist Walter Cannon in the early 1900s. But times are changing. Researchers are taking another look at the stress response in humans, and they are showing that "fight, flight, or freeze" is an incomplete list of the body's menu of options.

One of those researchers is Stephen Porges, the director emeritus of the Brain-Body Center of the College of Medicine at the University of Illinois–Chicago. His paradigm-breaking studies are what first identified a third branch of the autonomic nervous system: the smart vagus. The smart vagus is an evolutionarily newer pathway than the sympathetic or

parasympathetic nervous systems. While amphibians, reptiles, and fish have the older responses, only mammals have a
smart vagus in addition to the first two.

From an evolutionary perspective, the appearance of
the smart vagus went hand in hand with the appearance of
mammals and their increased social complexity and interde-
pendence. Until the evolution of mammals, the world was
populated by creatures that are less dependent on one another
for survival. For them, the sympathetic fight-or-flight response and the parasympathetic freeze response are adequate
to help them cope with the world. Have you ever wondered
why turtles lay piles of eggs and fish release large clumps of
roe? The primary reason for producing a large number of
offspring is to increase the odds that any one of them will
survive to reproduce. Young turtles, fish, and many other
nonmammalian creatures have no psychological or physical
need to be cuddled and fed by a parent; they leave the nest to
fend for themselves immediately after birth. They are born
with a complete set of instincts for hunting, eating, and hiding. They've got everything they need to survive in their
habitats . . . except size. Unfortunately, in their turtle-eat-fish
world, size matters. A lot. The only hope for the ultimate
survival of these premammalian species is to mass-produce
young and to hope that a few escape predation and survive into adulthood to reproduce. Though it has worked for
millennia, it is not a particularly efficient system for the prop-
agation of a species.

Mammals are different. Our reproduction efforts are more

efficient, in the sense that we produce fewer children, and those children have better odds of survival. One of the hallmarks of this system is a mammal baby's dependence on others for growth and development. A baby not only needs food and water, but also cuddling, cooing, and other stimulating contact with adults in order to grow and thrive. While turtles, fish, and frogs are born with instincts to manage the world on their own, mammals are born with a complete set of instincts to reach out to others. If you watch a newborn baby closely, you can see some of these instincts at work. The rooting reflex keeps an infant's neck and mouth turned toward the mother, searching for a breast for comfort and food; the Moro reflex causes an infant's arms to reach out, as if in a hug, when they are being put down. These instincts are vitally important, because a newborn mammal is not able to survive on his own without the help of a parent or older group member to care for him.

It appears that as mammals evolved and life on Earth became more socially complex, there was a need—or perhaps the opportunity—to use social connections as a way to moderate stress. Thus you and I have a smart vagus, a nerve that arises from the tenth cranial nerve at the base of the skull and heads north, where it links with some of the muscles of facial expression, speech, swallowing, and hearing. (Yes, hearing involves muscles—tiny ones—in your inner ear.) When you get input from other people's faces and voices telling you that these people are safe, the smart vagus sends a message to the sympathetic and parasympathetic nervous systems, telling them to turn off. In effect, the smart vagus says, "I'm with friends and everything is going to be okay. You don't need to fight, flee, or freeze right now." The smart vagus is one reason we feel less stress when we're around people we trust.

When you feel safe, the smart vagus also lets your muscles do the motor work that's necessary for engaging with the people around you. Your eyelids and eyebrows lift, so that your face becomes more open. The muscles of your inner ear tense, preparing you to hear the conversation. Without thinking about it, you look directly into the eyes of the people you're talking with. Your expression is animated, accurately reflecting your emotional response to the situation. This is a nerve that works to sustain social relationships, letting you send and receive emotional information that brings you closer to others and helps you feel calmer. Now *that's* smart.

In an ideal relational world, your autonomic nervous system automatically reads the environment and responds by activating the smart vagus when you are safe, the sympathetic nervous system when you are in danger, and the parasympathetic nervous system when your life is being threatened. But when your smart vagus isn't working well, you're less able to accurately interpret other people's intentions. Without the smart vagus doing its job, you can't see or hear other people as well, and you're at risk of misinterpreting their expressions. You don't make eye contact as easily, and your own facial expression becomes flatter, which increases the chances that you'll be seen as hostile or uncaring. Imagine how other people respond to your face when it looks closed off or angry.

If the smart vagus feels that other people are unsafe, it automatically shuts down.

It stops sending inhibitory messages to the sympathetic and parasympathetic nervous systems, allowing them to let loose with a stress response. If you're actually in danger, those stress responses are useful. But if you are around safe people *whom your nervous system has misread as unsafe*, imagine how problematic the feelings of the fight-or-flight response become. You get the familiar feelings of stress: elevated heart rate, sweaty palms, dry mouth, and fuzzy brain. You might not actually hit someone, but you may start an argument. Or you might perform the social equivalent of flight. (Have you ever zoned out during an uncomfortable conversation?) A parasympathetic freeze response is usually reserved for seriously life-threatening events, but in rare cases people who have experienced significant trauma at the hands of others can experience a partial shutdown in social situations. This goes way beyond a case of jitters; these folks literally can't speak or move.

In the case of Brooke, her smart vagus was off duty and her sympathetic nervous system was up and running as she entered the office party. Few people relish the idea of going to a cocktail party where they don't know a soul, but Brooke suffered from more than garden-variety butterflies. Brooke had a genetic tendency toward an overreactive stress response. In fact, both her mother and her mother's mother were anxious worriers who often preferred small, intimate groups to large crowds. These adults, however, were also capable of showing Brooke love and support. Both of these forces—anxiety and love—informed the way Brooke's autonomic nervous system responded to interpersonal interactions. She didn't have what neuroscientists call *good vagal tone*. Her smart vagus didn't always work as well as it should have, making it harder for her to navigate social situations. She tended to feel threatened by people she didn't know well, even when their intentions were friendly or neutral. And so, after spending a week in dread of the event, and without a friend's comforting presence, she was unable to read the smiling faces of the people around her as welcoming. To Brooke, those faces looked mocking and unreceptive. Her smart vagus, unable to sense that the environment was safe, failed to send a calming message to the sympathetic nervous system. Brooke didn't actually flee the party, but she did hide on the sidelines.

Brooke was unable to accurately read the expressions of strangers, but fortunately for her, her smart vagus wasn't completely broken. It was still able to respond to the presence of a friend. When Pete arrived and wished Brooke happy holidays, the vibrations from his kind, familiar voice traveled through space into her ear, moving the minuscule muscles that stimulated her smart vagus nerve. Almost immediately, she felt a wave of relief. Without thinking, her eyes scanned his smiling face and she responded with a delighted grin. As the muscles around her mouth and eyes tightened, they, too, stimulated her smart vagus. Instantaneously, the smart vagus sent an inhibitory message to both her sympathetic and parasympathetic nervous systems. She no longer had the urge to flee. She was safely in a conversation with Pete about fly-fishing. Not coincidentally, the other partygoers started to look friendlier—and she looked more receptive to them.

All in all, Brooke's social anxiety was fairly moderate. A friendly interaction could interrupt its loop. There are people who have it much worse. These are people with seriously poor vagal tone, sometimes because of genetic misfortune, but more often because their nervous system was shaped by an environment that was chronically threatening.

The human nervous system is shaped from infancy. A baby's life is full of routine stressors—hunger, sleepiness, wet diapers, sudden noises—that signal discomfort or danger and stimulate her sympathetic nervous system. Ideally, when a baby cries in distress, her caregivers respond supportively. They change her diaper, offer milk, or hold the baby tightly and rock her from side to side. This attuned adult–child relationship causes the baby's brain to release neurochemicals, like serotonin and endogenous opioids, that lessen the feeling of the threat. The baby's fear is soothed. Not only does the baby learn to associate her caregiver with safety, the experience helps her smart vagus become better connected with the parts of her brain that recognize safe faces, safe smells, safe noises, and so on. The multiple senses associated with a healthy relationship are eventually coded into the baby's nervous system. The regulatory pathway between the smart vagus and the sympathetic nervous system grows stronger and stronger. The result: human connection can now modulate the baby's stress response. The sympathetic and parasympathetic nervous systems can be soothed, or completely turned off, when the baby is in the presence of caring family and friends. The baby's sympathetic and parasympathetic nervous systems learn *not* to fire unless there is a real threat. The baby grows up with the ability to accurately distinguish between danger and safety, and she wants to seek out healthy human relationships.

This process of strengthening the smart vagus is one that continues throughout a child's life, into adulthood. If you have a terrible week at work, you may realize that you'll feel better if you have dinner with a friend Friday night. At the restaurant, you share the trials of the week, and your friend is appalled on your behalf. Your friend shares her own hard news: her mother has been diagnosed with a chronic illness. You cry together and laugh together, and at the end of the evening, you part ways. Not only do you feel better, the stimulation to your smart vagus has given it a fine tuning. Every time you share and receive comfort, your smart vagus becomes faster and more efficient at sending its chemical signals.

But what happens when the smart vagus develops within chaotic, disconnected, frightening circumstances? When a baby is repeatedly exposed to distress and is not soothed, her sympathetic nervous system is constantly stimulated. Her smart vagus doesn't learn to associate human relationships with comfort and safety. Her brain doesn't learn that there are times when the stress response can be turned off. She grows up hyperalert to danger, unable to relax even when she is safe, unable to enjoy other people even when their intentions are kind.

Infancy is the most significant time for brain development, but believe me: in a chronically dangerous environment, the smart vagus of an older child or adult will suffer.

If you are in constant danger because of a scary home situation, a violent neighborhood, or a war, your brain has a rational response—stay on high alert. Your sympathetic nervous system will flip to the On position, and depending on the intensity and consistency of the threat, it may more or less stay there. Your heart will race; your lungs will expand to take in more oxygen; and the blood vessels in your arms and limbs will dilate so more blood can flow through them. This way, you'll be prepared to fight or flee whenever the danger presents itself. If things are really bad, your parasympathetic nervous system might be preparing to bring on a freeze. But your body's nervous system is designed to respond to threats in short spurts, not twenty-four hours a day. Under extreme, chronic stress your body begins to break down. There's a greater risk of heart disease, illness, insomnia, depression . . . the list goes on. In fact, cortisol, the very chemical your body unleashes to counter the stress response, will damage brain cells needed for memory when it's released for too long.

The near-constant activation of the stress response is like exercise for your fight, flight, or freeze pathways. They become stronger and faster. At the same time, your smart vagus doesn't get the opportunity for a good workout. Eventually it will lose its good tone and become weak—leaving you with a loud and hypersensitive set of stress responses that perceives other people as basically dangerous and unkind, no matter what the reality. That's a tragedy, because we are built to use safe relationships as a way of reducing stress. Without this ability, we may look more independent, but in reality we are weaker and sicker. Happily, there are plenty of ways to improve the tone of your smart vagus. Later in the book, I'll describe these methods in detail.

A Is for Accepted: The Dorsal Anterior Cingulate Cortex

In 2003, three scientists at UCLA invited a series of volunteers to participate in an online game of catch called Cyberball.[1] The volunteer would arrive at the lab and, from inside a functional MRI scanner, begin playing the game. Things would start amicably enough, with the volunteer and researchers tossing the "ball" back and forth. So far, so good. But as things went on, the volunteer was gradually excluded from the game. No one explained to the volunteer why he or she wasn't receiving the ball anymore. No one even acknowledged that anything odd was going on. Eventually, the subject was completely left out as the other players tossed the ball among themselves.

Compared to other forms of social exclusion, like being beaten up on a playground or being snubbed because you look different from everyone else, getting inexplicably dropped from a game of Cyberball is pretty tame. But the researchers, Naomi Eisenberger and Matthew Lieberman, discovered that even this mild degree of social exclusion activated a specific part of the brain, the dorsal anterior cingulate cortex.

The dorsal anterior cingulate cortex, or dACC, is a small strip of the brain deep in the frontal cortex and part of a complex alarm system that—until this experiment—was primarily known for picking up the distress of physical pain. Walk into the corner of the kitchen table? The dACC activates. Catch your fingers in a drawer? That's your dACC, howling *Make this horrible feeling stop.*

So it was a surprise when the dACC lit up in response, not to being kicked or pinched, but to being left out. Remember, the volunteers weren't experiencing any physical harm. They were simply being excluded. The more emotionally distressed the volunteer was by the exclusion, the more activated the dACC became. The study's conclusion: to our brains, the pain of social rejection is the same as the pain from a physical injury or illness. That our major alarm system fires as a result of both physical pain and social pain is a measure of how important it is for us to be included—and how damaging it is to feel left out.

In our tough, hypercompetitive, gut-it-out culture, it is standard practice for some therapists to treat the pain of rejection or loneliness by encouraging the patient to become more emotionally independent. But when health professionals hear about this study that links social pain with physical pain, they tend to rethink this strategy. That's because the helping professions know to take physical pain seriously. Chronic physical pain is known to have significant medical consequences: it engages the stress response and causes depression, anxiety, and physical health problems. Imagine a person in extreme physical pain who visits an emergency room for help. Doctors might disagree about the best course of action, but most would try to treat both the pain itself as well as the underlying cause. No true medical professional would ever dream of dismissing this person's distress by saying, "We're going to reparent you so that you're less needy." After Cyberball, it seems incredibly cruel to do the same to someone who is suffering from social pain. Instead, it makes more sense to honor the pain and to help the person make healthy connections—because belonging to a group is, for all of us, more than one of life's fun perks. It's a biological requirement.

To understand why the dACC lights up when we're left out, let's look a little more closely at what we know about physical pain. In an interesting job share, your nerves register pain's noxious physical sensation, while your dACC registers how distressed you are by that sensation. The dACC is like a fire alarm that goes off when it senses smoke, warning you to get out of a burning house—except that this alarm goes off when you feel pain, telling you that you've got to do something about an injury. Without this alarm, you might not care enough to stop your hike through the woods and notice that your ankle hurts. Without that information, you might not see the blood that's gushing from a cut, and then you wouldn't know to stanch the flowing blood or to clean the wound. In other words, suffering from the sensation of pain gives you information that helps you preserve your physical well-being and even your life. On rare occasions, when a person has severe chronic pain whose underlying cause cannot be cured, a neurosurgeon may perform a cingulotomy, which is the surgical removal of the portion of the dACC associated with the distress of pain. What is so remarkable about this surgery is that afterward, the person still feels the physical sensation of pain but no longer feels bothered by it. Having a cingulotomy is like disconnecting your wailing smoke detector: you still have pain, but without the distress alarm, you might not have the impetus to seek out the source of the pain and stop it.

The fact that this same area of the dACC also registers the stress of social disconnection was revelatory to scientists, but I imagine our cave-people ancestors would find this discovery a no-brainer. Feeling distress from social pain was a way to alert them to the terribly risky condition of being alone. In a group, they could share information about food sources or team up to fight a mammoth. Alone, they were at high risk of starvation or being gored. And consider the experiment performed in the 1950s by the American psychologist Harry Harlow, who presented baby monkeys with two mother surrogates: a bare wire surrogate that provided food, or a surrogate that did not offer food but was covered with a soft cloth. The monkeys preferred the soft surrogate. For primates—and that includes you and me—there is a powerful

internal drive toward physical closeness, and it's more powerful than our drive for food. That biological need for connection is expressed, partly, in the behavior of the dACC.

When we respect our need for connection, we know to
pay attention to the distress call of the dACC. When we feel
isolated or excluded, we should be able to say, "This feels
awful. I need to do something about this!"—and then apply
our energies to the problem. We can reach out to dependable
friends. Where necessary, we can mend relational rifts or reconnect after long, sometimes awkward separations. We can
let our discomfort propel us to figure out why we're not included in the group, and then either change our behavior or
change the company we seek.

But when we adhere to the idea that it's healthier to be
separate and independent, we have a different reaction to the
brain's distress signal. Instead of listening to it, we try to
suppress it. We say, "I'm an idiot for feeling this way! I'm a
grown person; I shouldn't need anyone!" or "I'll just grin and
bear it." This is like hearing your smoke detector go off and
saying, "Well, I guess I just have to get used to that horrible
sound." You ignore the *cause* of the alarm. Meanwhile, your
house smolders.

I worry about what's happening to our brains in a world
that does not put a priority on connection. As humans, we are
blessed and cursed with the ability to form abstract thoughts
and an enormous capacity to remember past events. These
two characteristics of the human brain can enhance our enjoyment of life. You use these capacities when you conjure up

a fantasy about the date you are about to go on; or when you imagine an afternoon laughing by the pool with your best friends; or when you anticipate a loving reunion with your family after a long business trip away from home. Of course, you never really know how any interaction with another person will go. Essentially, you're making stuff up all the time, based on your past experiences.

The problem comes when you live in a culture that doesn't support healthy relationships or teach people how to make strong connections. Anyone who has a history of repeated social exclusion will use those painful experiences as a template for imagining the future. You expect more exclusion, and you will probably interpret your social encounters according to this expectation. The more you're left out, the more the experience of being left out is knitted into your neural pathways. Instead of anticipating happy reunions and pleasant social events, you tend to assume that you'll be rejected. And when *this* is the case, your dACC is almost always at least a little bit activated. This is especially problematic when people experience rejection and abuse in childhood, a time when their brains are creating their initial pathways for relationship. They live with an alarm system that is constantly ringing. The nerve pathway that is supposed to help them stay connected becomes a nerve pathway that keeps them frightened and apart.

One of my favorite movies, *Good Will Hunting*, illustrates how past relationships can create an overactive dACC. The lead character, Will, was born and raised in gritty South

Boston (back before the townies moved there and spruced it up). Will is an Einstein-level math genius working as a janitor in the hallowed halls of MIT during the day and hanging out with his townie buddies in the evening. He meets a Harvard girl, Skylar, at a local bar, and charms her with his intellect, humor, and good looks. As their relationship gets more intimate, Skylar tries to deepen their commitment—and Will flips out. He rages at her, yelling while revealing his childhood history of neglect and abuse. (I'll go out on a limb here and suggest that screaming is rarely an effective way to communicate vulnerability.) At the peak of his outburst, Will lifts up his shirt and reveals a long red scar on his torso where one of his foster parents had stabbed him. It's clear that by exposing the physical evidence of his deepest wounds, Will is not inviting Skylar to be closer to him; he's aggressively trying to scare her away for good. He caps the scene by telling Skylar that he doesn't love her and storming out of the room.

You might know someone like Will; you might even be someone like Will. His relational template—which can also be called his controlling image, because of the way it significantly controls his adult life—was formed early and reinforced repeatedly by severe beatings, frequent abandonment, neglect, and poverty. For all of us, early environments are the shapers of our young neural pathways, including the distress meter, the dACC. For Will, and for many other survivors of severe abuse or neglect, the dACC has linked intimacy with the threat of abandonment and physical pain. This is the brain's equivalent of a DEFCON 1 scenario. In response, your ability to think gets tossed like nonessential personnel while your brain unleashes its most potent weapon: a cascade of terror and survival instincts. When that happens, a person trying to get closer is indistinguishable from a person moving in for the kill.

Traumatized people are not the only ones with overactive dACCs. Milder experiences with rejection also have lingering effects. Even if you had an ideally loving childhood and rejection-free adolescence, you're still living in a culture that measures success by how little you need other people and by whether you've battled your way to the top. Sure, we *know* that we're supposed to be nice to other people, and that everyone matters. But we still socialize around hierarchy and stratification. Children very early on learn their ABCs—but they also pick up from the adults around them that it's vital to sort the smartest from the dumbest and the fastest from the slowest, to know which kids are shipped from the inner city to the suburbs for a better education and which kids can walk to the same school from their very large house. In our culture, extreme competitiveness is at the core of child rearing and brain building. I'm not disparaging normal, healthy competition here. (Put me on a basketball court, and I will *take you down* . . . but then we'll go out afterward for cake.) I'm talking about the kind of competition that is really judgmental, the kind that becomes the basis for deciding who is worthy of love and acceptance, the kind that has everyone worrying that it's only a matter of time before they're voted off the island.

In a competitive, judgmental, unaccepting environment,

everyone's relational templates are distorted, and everyone's dACC is reactive to some degree. You can see the proof in the adults who have an exaggerated need to control the in-crowd at work or social activities. These people may act like they are kings or queens of the hill, but the harder they try to make sure they are "in" by leaving others out, the more anxious they become about being pushed out of the "in" group. If these folks weren't so afraid of candor, they would tell you that being on the bottom of the pile is so excruciating that they will avoid it at all costs—but being alone at the top is pretty destructive, too.

At the other extreme is the person who moves seamlessly into the outsider role, with no expectation of being welcome or included in any group. The first kind of person carries the weight of rage; the other carries the weight of shame. Both emotions go hand in hand with feeling unworthy of inclusion in the larger human community. And both are the cause and result of social exclusion—and an overactive dACC.

R Is for Resonant: The Mirroring System

Resonance is the deep nonverbal connection between our bodies and brains that allows our hands to feel warm when another person rubs his together, or to sense a friend's sorrow even before she tells you about it. It's the sense of "getting" another person, of instinctively knowing him. The neural basis for resonance is what Rizzolatti and his team first stumbled on to when they discovered that a monkey's brain internally mimicked the action of a researcher lifting his arm.

The mirroring system that creates resonance is the third C.A.R.E. pathway, and its story becomes even more fantastic when you consider the role it plays in understanding what another person is saying. The next time you have ten minutes, a clean pencil, and a nearby friend, try this experiment. It was designed by Paula Niedenthal, of the Niedenthal Emotions Laboratory at the University of Wisconsin–Madison, to highlight the important role of the mirroring system in understanding each other.[2]

Sit comfortably across from each other and think of a detailed, emotional story. The first listener should place a pencil or pen horizontally in his mouth and keep it there while the speaker tells his story. Once the story is told, switch roles.

Did either of you notice a difference in listening while the pen engaged the muscles of your mouth? I use this exercise with workshop participants, and I hear a similar set of responses every time. The first few comments usually focus on how ridiculous and distracted the speakers felt as they tried to communicate with someone who has a pen in his mouth. When pushed to think about the content of what they heard when they were listeners, the reaction is usually unanimous— it is more difficult to understand what is being said when the muscles in your face are busy holding the pen. For most of us, this is a strange and unexpected response. After all, the pen was not stuck in your ears. What in the world is going on here?

Stephen Wilson was a research student at UCLA when he began studying the connection between speaking and listening, using functional brain imaging to see the brain in action. He discovered that the exact same part of the brain was activated when his research subjects were listening as when they were speaking.[3] In another study looking at the overlap between speaking and listening, the German neurologist Ingo Meister used another new technique called *transcranial magnetic stimulation* to effectively turn off the speech center of a person's brain. He found that when the motor neurons controlling speech are turned off, people have difficulty understanding what they are hearing.[4] Apparently, when in conversation, internally mirroring the other person's speech is essential to understanding it.

So what happens when your face is really paralyzed? Let's say rather than placing a pencil in your mouth to disable your ability to make expressions, you have a condition that prohibits you from moving the muscles of your face. People born with Moebius syndrome, a rare disorder that affects the cranial nerves, present researchers with an opportunity to explore this question in real life. People with Moebius syndrome live with a frozen face and are found to have a more difficult time communicating their emotions to other people. Given how much we count on facial expressions in showing our feelings to others, this is no big shock. What has been surprising to researchers is that Moebius syndrome also makes it more difficult to read other people's emotions. Just as holding a pencil between your teeth keeps your brain from mimicking another person's speech, paralysis of the facial muscles prevents people with Moebius syndrome from internally copying other people. Because this mimicking is key to understanding what a person is hearing, victims of this disorder have a much more difficult time understanding other people. People who get Botox treatments for facial wrinkles also have a harder time reading others.[5] Because injections of Botox temporarily paralyze the muscles, they aren't able to perform internal mimicking in the same the way they are used to.

Your brain mirrors far more than other people's movements. After the Rizzolatti monkey study, a number of studies showed that the mirroring system works on a profound level. If you see another person experiencing pain, your brain mimics the experience. When you watch another person smile or frown, both of your brains will activate in the same regions as that person's, although your brain activity won't be as intense. Your mirror system activates even when another person simply gives a hint that he is about to do something. If, say, you're in line at Starbucks and the man in front of you begins to move his arm, you may simply "know" that he is about to point to a slice of lemon cake—even though he's not actually pointing yet—and that's because your brain is copying the experience and using that information to read his actions and emotions, and anticipate what he might do. And other people are doing the same with you.

The mirroring system appears to be a crucial element in the complex act of empathy. Once your mirror system registers information about what another person is doing or the feeling she is expressing, that information passes through the insula, a small strip of tissue that lies deep within the brain and helps attach content to feeling states. The mirroring experience becomes a feeling you have in connection with another person's feeling.

Of course, there's a limit. We don't copy every action we witness in another person, or feel every single thing that everyone else around us is feeling. That would be exhausting and paralyzing. A world of unfiltered emotions would be a nightmare! Fortunately, for most of us, biology has, again, saved the day by creating a *super mirroring system* as an integral part of the grand design to read others.

The super mirroring system acts like the brakes on an idling car. These days, cars with automatic transmissions have a baseline level of movement when you pull up to a stoplight. If all you do is take your foot off the gas, the car moves forward. If you want to keep the car from moving, you have to put your foot on the brake. Likewise, the classical mirroring system is constantly picking up the feelings and actions of people around you—and sometimes you need to put a brake on that activity and keep yourself in a more neutral state. That's when the super mirroring system steps in. Thanks to the super mirroring system, if you see someone crying, you do not necessarily break out in sobs; if you see someone reaching for the coffee shop pastry, your arm does not have to reach out, too.

Marco Iacoboni, the UCLA psychiatrist and author, believes that the super mirroring system has a regulatory, inhibitory impact on our classical mirroring system so that we do not physically act out every action or feeling we see in others. In collaboration with Itzhak Fried, a researcher whose studies of epilepsy involved placing electrodes on individual brain cells, Iacoboni is beginning to map the super mirroring system in the frontal lobe of the brain. Whether or not you actually enact a movement or simply know that another has made the same movement is dependent on how the two systems—the classical mirroring system and super mirroring system—interact. The classical mirroring system fires both when you move your arm and when you watch someone across the room move his arm. The inhibitory, super mirroring system is more active when you watch someone move his arm, however, and less active when you are moving your arm.

My experience with a client, Jessica, shows how both systems work together to bring about an empathic response. Jessica texted me the night before her therapy appointment to tell me that her boyfriend of one year, the man she thought she would marry—the man *everyone* thought she would marry— had broken up with her. Ray had been unusually distant for about two weeks, but Jessica figured that with the holidays coming up and with his family in town, he was simply busy and less available. She tried to reassure herself that things would be back to normal once the New Year started. They met up for what Jessica thought would be an ordinary dinner, and he broke up with her on the spot. The text read simply: *Ray just broke up with me. I am devastated!*

When I saw her in my waiting room the next morning,

my mirroring system was immediately activated. As my eyes registered her red, sad-looking eyes and the downward turn of her mouth, neurons in my prefrontal cortex were stimulated so that internally my own state mimicked her misery. Nerve cells in my somatosensory cortex re-created the state of having itchy, puffy, crying-all-night eyes. As my insula relayed the information to my own visceral system, I felt a tightening in my stomach and a heaviness in my chest. This empathetic experience of Jessica's pain happened in an instant.

Fortunately, my super mirroring system (a therapist's best friend) was also activated, enabling me to have a taste of what my client was feeling—but *just* a taste. As Jessica sat and wept, head in her hands, I felt a tear well up in my own eye, but I never got close to sobbing myself. This ability to modulate is crucial to maintaining healthy connections. Think about it. If we were all simply mimicking everything all the time, there would be a single feeling that traveled through humanity in a gigantic wave. Thankfully, that doesn't happen.

When the mirroring system fires in empathic response, it is not an exact duplicate of another person's experience, nor is it a complete merger of feelings. Jessica's sadness, however, was strong enough and clear enough for us to be joined through an empathic connection. Just as a fish knows how to turn in unison with the rest of its school, Jessica and I instinctively knew how to move closer together in this magical, mutual moment. It's not just emotional; it's biological, down to our nerve cells. Physically, emotionally, and neurologically, we were in sync. It was a reminder to both of us that, as human beings, we are never alone in the world.

Unfortunately, the separation-individuation model of human development doesn't leave a lot of space for thinking about the mirroring system and warm, connected closeness. It was not too long ago that mental health providers were taught that empathy did not belong in the therapy hour. The idea was that empathy was a contagion that would distort the real work of therapy—which was, supposedly, helping a person identify mental blocks preventing him from "standing on his own two feet." Now many therapists identify empathy as *the* most important ingredient in a healthy healing relationship. But you still see the old attitude in the idea that we're not supposed to need other people to share in our happiness or heartache, or that healthy individuals should be able to avoid "catching" other people's feelings. You certainly see it in our competitive day-to-day environment, in which we tend to view other people as adversaries, not potential friends, and everyone is under near-constant stress. In our ideal of success, you are admired for your ability to do what is necessary without considering the impact on others. To unwind from the tension, people play violent video games or watch violent television shows.

This environment actively undermines the natural physiology of connection. In a competitive, visually violent world, you're exposed to so much pain that the only way to thrive is to ignore the signals that your mirroring system sends you about other people's feelings, actions, and intentions. It's true that mirroring activities happen involuntarily, but it's possible to consciously reject the signals that other people send you. Over time, it's even possible to develop the capacity to dissociate from your own body, which is a bigger version of paralyzing your facial muscles by holding a pencil in your mouth—it makes it harder for you to decode the feelings of others. When you are disconnected from your body, you also miss out on the sensations that signal your own feeling states. Years ago, I treated a woman who had been physically abused as a child. Over the years, she learned to decouple her bodily messages from her thoughts, as a way to protect herself from feeling pain. She had so effectively ignored her basic body signals for so long, however, that as an adult, she had no idea what it felt like to be hungry. That slight ache you feel in the sternum when you wake up in the morning? You and I know this to be hunger—but my client barely registered the feeling. When she *did* notice the feeling, she thought it was a stomachache. As a result, she rarely ate in the mornings, and the rest of the day she barely ate enough to keep herself going. She had to relearn how to focus on her body in order to understand messages that she should have read instinctively.

Whenever an uncomfortable empathic message—like pain—comes through, you can choose to withdraw from it. Do this often enough, and your mirroring system takes a hit. Because the mirroring system is made of nerve cells throughout your brain, especially in the areas that govern action, sensation, and feeling, the system can thrive only when it's used repeatedly. As you'll see in the next chapter, complex neural pathways are made stronger by being "wired together"—by being stimulated over and over. It's this wiring together of different brain regions that forms the 3-dimensional experience of another person's world. It makes the information you get clearer and more complex, which means that the empathic response you feel is more likely to be in tune with what the person is actually feeling. Without frequent stimulation, the pathways between the neurons become weaker and less able to carry signals. Our complex mirror nerve system needs to be stimulated in order for us to maintain this gift of reading each other.

Is it inevitable that we will lose our ability to communicate and read one another as we interact increasingly through technology? I don't think so, but it is necessary to educate children and adults about the essential role of the mirroring system in our human interactions and teach them how to keep this part of their nervous systems robust. As I sit typing this chapter in Panera, I see and hear groups engaged in good old-fashioned conversation. Elderly men and women are gathered at a large table, laughing, talking, drinking coffee, eating muffins—and stimulating their mirroring system. Another group of coworkers is discussing a work project, two of them huddled over their computers. They are typing ideas, talking, laughing, drinking coffee—and stimulating their mirroring systems. My kids are now at school. In a typical day, they might be working in small groups in science lab and learning how to divvy up tasks and to cooperate in writing a report; sitting at lunch acting goofy with their friends; or asking teachers for help—in all these interactions, they are stimulating their mirroring systems. These human interactions are as ubiquitous as Apple products these days. What shapes us is not so much the devices we use, but the culture in which the device is placed. If, as a society, we value human connection as the center of our lives, and if we understand the need to stimulate our mirroring systems to maintain our ability to read others and to cooperate in groups, then the electronic world will follow.

E Is for Energetic: The Dopamine Reward System

On the fourth relational pathway, we meet up with dopamine, a neurotransmitter that makes our lives feel more gratifying. Like many of our neurotransmitters, dopamine plays a different role in our brains and bodies depending on which neural pathway it is traveling. The dopamine pathway that is most directly connected to relationships is the one that is involved in our brain's reward system. This pathway, known as the *mesolimbic pathway*, starts in the brain stem. It then sends projections to the amygdala, which is involved in feelings and emotions, and travels through the thalamus, which acts like a kind of relay station. The mesolimbic pathway ends in the orbitomedial prefrontal cortex, where some of the decision-making process takes place. The pathway then loops back to the brain stem and modulates the production of dopamine.

When dopamine is stimulated in this pathway, you feel good. Remember Jean Baker Miller's description of growth-fostering relationships as "zestful"? Dopamine gives you that zest; it can feel like a shot of warm, glowing, motivating energy. This is a system whose purpose is to reward healthy, growth-promoting activities—like eating well, having sex, and being in a good relationship—with a supply of dopamine that makes us feel great. The resulting feelings of elation make us want to participate in more of those healthy activities. It encourages the human population to do what's good for us.

It's a brilliant setup, but only when it works the way it's supposed to. In an ideal world, you're born with a brain that pairs human contact and dopamine. And then, in your first months and years, your early relationships are so rewarding and healthy that your dopamine system learns to connect relationships even more tightly with feeling good. In one study, the more dopamine receptors in the striatum (part of the forebrain), the better your social status and social support.[6] More dopamine, more interconnection.

But what happens to this pathway when a baby or child does not experience snuggly, supportive relationships? What happens to children who are raised to be fiercely "independent" above all else? To children raised to believe that counting on others throughout life makes them weak and vulnerable? In these children, relationships become disconnected from the dopamine reward system. Seen from the brain's perspective, this is a logical protective step: if relationships are threatening or seen as unhealthy, they should not be paired up with a rewarding boost of dopamine. These children become adults who simply don't get much pleasure from relationships. Instead of becoming energized by friendships—even good ones—they are drained and depleted by the interaction.

When the dopamine system is disconnected from healthy relationships, the brain looks for other ways to feel good—so it seeks out other ways to stimulate the dopamine system. Those "other ways" are familiar to all of us: overeating, drug and alcohol abuse, compulsive sex, shopping, risk-taking activities, gambling.

This is why you may have heard either dopamine or the mesolimbic pathway getting a bad rap. Recently it's been discovered that all drugs of addiction—and in fact all addictions, whether or not they're drug-based—stimulate the mesolimbic pathway and release dopamine. The more this pathway is repeatedly stimulated by a particular drug or activity, the more robust the addiction gets.

It's important to understand how a pathway that's meant in part to encourage healthy human connection can get hijacked to create drug addictions. Addictive drugs, such as cocaine, heroin, and marijuana, have a two-pronged attack on the central nervous system. A drug's first action on the body is unique to that drug. Cocaine produces its euphoria and grandiosity by stimulating the release of a large amount of the naturally occurring neurotransmitter norepinephrine. Heroin, on the other hand, works by imitating the effects of the body's naturally occurring opioids.

While the initial high a drug causes is compelling, it is the second action of addictive drugs, the stimulation of the dopamine reward system, that ultimately leads to addiction. With repeated use of a drug, the body adapts by either producing less dopamine or down-regulating its receptors. When this happens, you get less of a "hit," or reward, from the drug. Over time, tolerance develops so you need more of the drug to produce the same high. This double whammy of an altered mental state and stimulation of the dopamine reward system serves as the perfect storm for addiction.

Substance abuse may be the most well-known addiction, but it certainly is not alone. In reality, any activity done so repetitively that it gets in the way of other meaningful activities in life is an addiction. In a perversion of the dopamine pathway's original purpose, your brain learns to pair dopamine with activities that are incredibly *un*healthy. When the powerful chemistry of addiction sets in, humans are no different from rats in a lab that obsessively press a lever to receive stimulants even as they are starving to death. Producing dopamine trumps all other life-sustaining activities.

The science of addiction is specific and devastating. But in a way, we all seek out dopamine. We *all* live from one dopamine hit to another, and it's natural for us to want to feel good. What matters is the source of the dopamine. It can be as life affirming as drinking water or cuddling a newborn baby—or it can be as destructive as a drug addiction. But every single one of us craves dopamine. It is simply the nature of human physiology and the behavior of the dopamine reward system.

When we are under pressure to be highly separate, intensely independent individuals, we are at risk for cutting ourselves off from one of the primary healthy sources of dopamine. But it is possible to rewire your brain so that it can get more pleasure out of relationships—to crave human contact instead of unhealthy substitutes. The key, as Louis Cozolino writes in *The Neuroscience of Human Relationships*, is to understand that "healing involves reconnecting our dopamine reward system to relationships."[7] With practice and an understanding of how the dopamine system works, you can teach your brain to stop searching for dopamine in all the wrong places—and that the easiest way to feel better is to reach out to another safe human being.

The science is clear. Social disconnection stimulates our brain's pain pathways and our stress response systems, making it more likely we'll seek out unhealthy sources of dopamine. We also miss out on the richness of human experience, of the empathic connections that are intricately tied to the depth and breadth of feeling and emotion.

But there is plenty that you can do to nourish your neurological pathways for connection. If they are damaged, you can start to heal them. If they are neglected, you can cultivate them. And if they are stressed, you can soothe them. In the next chapter, I'll describe the science that is teaching us how to change our brains for the better.

Chapter 3

THE THREE RULES
OF BRAIN CHANGE

By now it should be clear that we are not as psychologically independent and separate as we've been led to believe. For better or worse, relationships reach deep inside our brains to shape how we feel, think, and react.

Ideally, our relationships are healthy and help us feel great—Calm, Accepted, Resonant, and Energetic. So great, in fact, that we crave *more* relationships, and we knit together a network of people who help us mature into even greater relational complexity. If that doesn't sound like you, well . . . welcome to the club, my friend. In a world that dismisses our biological need for warm, human connection, most of us have suffered through some pretty bad relationships or felt the chill of isolation. That means our brains have suffered, too. Instead of feeling Calm, Accepted, Resonant, and Energetic, you might feel any or all of the opposite: irritable, rejected, bewildered, and tired. You might even have the sense that you're just not good with people, or that you weren't built to enjoy relationships.

There is another perspective that needs to shift, and this is the idea that a history of difficult relationships can be traced to a fixed, unchangeable flaw in our personalities.

This is untrue. Both our genes and the environment will, over the years, write particular relational patterns into the brain—but they are not necessarily written onto our souls. It can be helpful to see these problems as nothing more than electrical impulses that, instead of following the four C.A.R.E. pathways for healthy relationships, go off track. With understanding and effort and support, it is possible to redirect those wayward impulses. We can shrink undesirable neural pathways that undermine our relationships and strengthen other pathways that are more beneficial. We can even grow neural connections that are completely new. These new or healthier pathways can help us do what we are designed to do: enjoy satisfying relationships in which we can grow.

Neurology Does a 180

Sally, a client who initially came to me because she had developed a habit of lying to her boyfriends, is a good example of how an adult can learn to change her brain, and how relationships are a vital part of that change.

My mother used to say to my siblings and me, "Why lie? The truth is far more interesting." This was not the case with Sally. Real life was almost never as interesting as her lies. If Sally didn't feel like going out on a Saturday night, she'd tell her boyfriend that she was going on a weekend trip . . . to London. If she was running late for a date, she'd say that her tires had been slashed. There were other kinds of lies, too: if Sally's boyfriend liked action movies, Sally—who preferred foreign films—would pretend to like them, too. Did Sally want to help her boyfriend finance a car? Let him move in without paying rent? Of course she did!

Flexibility is essential to relationships, perhaps especially romantic relationships. We have to be able to imagine each other's experiences of life and compassionately negotiate our different needs. But Sally was a relational contortionist who twisted herself like a pretzel to fit the desires of whatever man she happened to be dating. She wanted men to feel that she could perfectly suit their needs—that she would never be disagreeable, would never be late, and would never want to do anything different from what her boyfriend wanted to do. Sally's lies weren't just lies; they were her strategy for staying connected in her romantic relationships. They were also a source of dopamine, the neurotransmitter that creates a sense of pleasurable energy. When she told a whopper, she felt a rush of excitement—would she get caught this time?—as well as anticipation of tenderness from her boyfriend as he heard of her latest tragedy or her willingness to support his plans. But Sally's romances came to a predictable end: within a few months, she'd told so many lies and hidden so much of herself that the relationship was unsustainable. Sally came to me because she wanted to stop this pattern. But after more than a decade of advanced lying, could she change?

Common methods of addressing a problem like Sally's include the "you need to have more self-control" school of thought, which draws on the old separation-individuation model. The general idea is that Sally has to get a grip on herself and stop doing things that undermine her relationships. If she feels the impulse to lie, she should simply ignore that impulse, even if she has to white-knuckle her way through it until the temptation passes. There is some wisdom here, because self-control is an essential element of change. But this approach doesn't account for the complex role of relationships in Sally's problem, or the way that lying had become wired to the dopamine reward system in her brain. The self-control approach also doesn't take advantage of neurological methods of brain change. (For example, the neurochemicals produced by healthy relationships can help melt pathways for bad habits and solidify new pathways that are more desirable.) Not to mention that the self-control approach leads to a classically depressing circle: if Sally feels that the measure of her maturity is the ability to stand alone and control herself, she will feel like a childish failure if she gives in to temptation and tells a lie. Then she'll seek comfort in her most reliable source of dopamine—namely, telling some really impressive lies in order to elicit excitement and love.

Then again, some therapists might try to help Sally break her lying habit by looking at her present and past relationships. A psychodynamic therapist would probably try to understand her family history, for example, and talk about how Sally's parents had never accepted the true, real Sally—they'd preferred the false version she'd learned to present to them. There would likely be a lot of discussion about how she tended to choose boyfriends who were a little *too* comfortable having a woman meet all their needs. Most of all, there would be a big dose of understanding acceptance. These are wonderful qualities to bring into a healing, therapeutic relationship. However, they are not always enough to bring about brain change, and even when they are, that change can be a long time coming. Although I suspected that Sally's lying was connected to the nature of her past and present relationships, I worried that traditional talk therapy would not be enough to help her dig out of this entrenched habit.

Why are we stuck with only these two options—self-control and therapeutic acceptance—for changing habits and relational patterns? One reason is that most people, even therapists, aren't aware of the neuroscience of connection. Another reason is that for centuries, the brain was seen as fixed and unchangeable. Yet there is overwhelming evidence that the brain can change—that it is, in fact, always changing.

Your Brain Is Alive

Until recently, scientists could not actually see the brain or measure its components. Tucked away neatly inside the skull, its nature has been hidden. Scientists who were unable to witness the brain in action have struggled over the centuries to create models and theories to explain its enormous capacity. The brain has been compared to a chest of drawers with many discrete compartments; to a filing cabinet with folders that can be opened and closed; to the Wizard of Oz, controlling the city from behind his curtain; and to a supercomputer, endlessly performing operations along its circuits. All these analogies are to essentially inorganic, mechanical objects. These objects aren't alive. They don't grow and they don't change.

For the most part, scientists believed the same thing about the human brain, with one exception: childhood. It was believed that childhood was the only time that the brain could grow and adapt. A child soaks up signals from the internal and external environment and—for better or worse—the child's brain adapts to that environment. In a case that Antonio Battro documents in his book *Half a Brain Is Enough: The Story of Nico*, doctors removed the right lobe of a boy's brain in an attempt to treat his seizures. Despite Nico's loss of crucial brain tissue, he developed virtually without deficits. He developed not just the kind of functions associated with the left side of the brain, but musical and mathematical abilities as well—even though those functions are usually controlled by the brain's right side. Battro explains that the traditional explanation for how the boy's brain could compensate when half of it had been removed was that a child's brain is still developing during childhood.[1]

The old belief was that this kind of extreme compensation for a brain deficit or injury was possible—though rare—only while a child is still growing. As a child moves into puberty, scientists believed, the brain becomes fixed in place and no outside pressure can reshape it. No more growth, no more adaptation. At that point, if something from the outer world does damage the brain, that damage is mostly irreparable. To take a psychological example, children who grow up with unattuned, uninterested caregivers develop brains that result in behavior patterns reflecting hopelessness. According to the old model of brain development, such a child's only hope is early, caring intervention to reshape the brain. Without it, the child's emotional fate is sealed. Other physical and emotional traumas could carve their signatures into the young brain, too.

In an extension of the brain-as-hardware metaphor, it was also believed that the brain's destiny was to break down. Little by little, as it took the hits that befell it over the course of a normal lifetime, the brain's components would rust and short out. Or it could suffer a spectacular crash, with large parts of the brain going dark as the result of an accident, infection, or stroke. In this view, cells in the central nervous system are like pieces in a set of antique china; if you break one, there is nothing to do but sweep up the broken pieces and carry on as best you can with whatever is left intact.

No one believed that brain cells might be able to repair themselves or regenerate, or develop new connections among themselves. This depressing neurological "fact" had serious consequences for people who had injuries or illnesses that affected the brain. Until about fifteen years ago, it was standard for rehabilitation hospitals to aggressively treat people in the first few weeks or months after their injury, but once the brain swelling subsided and improvement plateaued, it was believed that nothing more could be done. Rehabilitation meant learning how to compensate for whatever deficits you'd developed. If you injured your visual cortex (the part of the brain usually associated with vision), it meant you had cortical blindness, period. If you lost function of your left arm, that arm would forever hang limp. Rehab therapists would teach you how to get around without seeing or how to get your groceries through the front door while using only your right arm. And if you had difficult relationships as a child, it was assumed that these relationships left an indelible scar on your capacity to connect.

Fortunately, this view of the brain can be now placed in the medical-history archives, filed away with other outdated ideas like bloodletting and black bile (the "humour" that Hippocrates thought caused cancer and other illnesses). Although the brain still needs protection, and I don't recommend knocking it around, your brain is not quite the fixed, fragile object we once thought it was. As you'll see throughout the book, you can use the rules of brain change to solve problems, repair your C.A.R.E pathways, and strengthen your relationships.

Brain Change Rule Number 1:
Use It or Lose It

A friend of mine developed tinnitus, a disorder in which your nerves "hear" a sound that is not there. She described the sound as a high-pitched noise that stayed in the background during the day, when she was distracted by work or her kids. When she lay down to sleep at night, however, the noise seemed to get louder. With fewer other sounds to compete with the noise, nighttime became a nightmare. After a few months she was chronically sleep deprived; eventually, she was depressed. Then her doctor told her about a new treatment, one that would use a principle called *competitive neuroplasticity* to weaken the area of her cortex that was producing the phantom sound. The treatment was time intensive: for a couple of hours a day, the doctor had my friend listen to music she loved but from which the pitch that matched the ringing sound was deleted. After the treatments, her tinnitus was dramatically reduced and no longer interfered with her ability to sleep at night. Slowly, her life regained its old, normal hectic form.

If you'd had tinnitus several years ago, you would have

been told that it was untreatable. It was in 1997 that a surge of discoveries about the brain began, discoveries that led straight to this treatment for tinnitus, along with therapies for other disorders that originate in the nervous system. These are treatments that let us rewrite our brain pathways. They are becoming more familiar in certain settings, especially the rehabilitation hospital and the occupational therapist's office. In other settings, including the psychotherapy office, they are not familiar enough. When your relational pathways aren't working in the way you'd like them to, it is possible to change them.

The watershed event in 1997 was a study by Peter Eriksson, a Swedish neuroscientist who proved that the adult human brain can grow new neurons. Until then, it was thought that the adult brain was like hair on a balding scalp: although it was natural to lose neurons as you aged, and not necessarily a sign of disease, you could never grow new ones. Eriksson's discovery had many implications, but one of its greatest effects was to throw open a door onto a new field of research. This field is called *neuroplasticity*; the idea is that the adult brain can be remolded and reshaped, much the way a soft plastic polymer can be pulled and pushed into shape. Suddenly, the hardware metaphors for the brain no longer fit the known facts. The brain is not fixed. It is more versatile and more resilient than anyone ever guessed. It is more alive.

Neural pathways are constantly responding to their environment. When you stimulate a brain pathway repeatedly, it grows stronger. It grows more myelin, allowing electrical impulses to travel faster along its length. More branches develop, making the path wider. (Seen through a microscope, a well-traveled neural pathway has so many branches that it looks wild and bushy, like Einstein's hair.) Brain pathways also compete with one another for space, so as you use a particular pathway more and more frequently, other pathways die off. This leaves fewer alternative pathways for the brain's electrical impulses to travel. Instead of dispersing themselves along several different smaller paths, more impulses run together along the well-traveled one.

But if neurons are starved of stimuli for long enough and if your brain does not sense a demand for their use, they can wither away. If you could look at the brain of a person who's lost the use of a body part to amputation or paralysis, you'd see that the brain's "map" no longer features roads and pathways for that part. The area those pathways used to travel is not empty, however. It is grown over by other, nearby pathways that are taking advantage of the abandoned real estate.

This is why the tinnitus treatment works. The competitive sound forces the patient off the old pathway so that it's not used so repetitively; it also encourages a new, alternative pathway to grow. Rehabilitation specialists harness the use-it-or-lose-it rule with new protocols for stroke victims. Instead of merely teaching them how to compensate for lost function, they also will stimulate the neural pathways for the disabled body part by working it over and over.

The "use it or lose it" rule is also at work when people get stuck in relational patterns. You can see this when a long-married couple has "forgotten" how to talk about their problems without bickering and sniping: the neural pathways for these habits have, over the course of their marriage, become hardened and inflexible. Or when a woman always shows up with a date who drinks too much. For a person like this, there is probably a psychological tug of familiarity at work—maybe her parents had similar attributes—but there is a neurological factor, too. A neural track was laid down in her brain in childhood, creating a template that associates important relationships with alcohol. As she follows that template as an adult, and continues to follow it, she wears a neurological groove, replaying one set of preferences and behaviors over and over, until the alternative paths weaken from disuse. You also see "use it or lose it" when someone undergoes what looks like a significant change of temperament. A quiet person moves to a big city and becomes bolder; a selfish person undergoes a hardship and becomes more empathic. The changed circumstances force changes in the brain pathways.

Sally, my client who lied to her boyfriends, had a fast, strong neural pathway for lying that had been reinforced over years of repetition. Our work together would run in the same direction as the therapy for tinnitus. We wanted to intentionally weaken the path of her habit. At the same time, we'd stimulate some alternative pathways—relational ones—in the hope that they'd grow strong enough to compete with the old one.

Brain Change Rule Number 2: Neurons That Fire Together, Wire Together

The second rule of brain change is **Neurons that fire together, wire together.** Like people, neurons are stronger in groups. When neurons that are close to each other repeatedly fire at the same time, they will eventually link up and form part of a neural network or pathway. A neuron is made up of a nucleus, axons, and dendrites. Axons send messages toward other neurons, and dendrites receive other neurons' messages. It's as if axons and dendrites reach out from separate neurons and hold hands. (Their handholding is done across a gap called a *synapse*, into which neurotransmitters release chemical messengers that are passed from neuron to neuron.) In an immature nervous system, this handholding looks clean and simple. You can imagine that Neuron A holds hands with Neuron B, which holds hands with Neuron C—sort of like children playing a game of Red Rover. But with stimulation and the passage of time, neurons grow more axons and dendrites. They reach out to hold hands with many neurons, forming complex neural networks.

The direction that these pathways take, and their degree of complexity, is based partly on the DNA of the individual neurons. But the new field of epigenetics tells us that the expression of DNA is profoundly affected by the stimulation your neurons receive from the environment. DNA aside, your neurons and neural pathways are also directly shaped by environmental triggers. Consider the track that leads from the motor cortex of the brain to the right index finger. We're all born with this track. As a child who is studying piano repeatedly stimulates that track, it grows stronger, with more axons and dendrites—that's the "use it or lose it" rule in effect. But those axons and dendrites don't simply wave around with nothing to do. They reach out and hold hands with other neurons; in "neurospeak," they recruit neurons from nearby pathways. Brain scans of concert pianists show that the neural networks for their fingers are richly interconnected; the axons and dendrites of the relevant neurons have grown together so tightly that the whole hand operates as one unified part, rather than as five separate fingers plus palm and wrist. This interconnectedness results from the repeated stimulation of the different parts of the hand at the same time. Over the years, the hand's neural network recruits even more neurons into its pathway. The nerve cells themselves will be slightly larger because they have each grown so many branches, but a thicker pathway also results from the pathway finding more and more friends, all joining into this neural network. If a pathway like this is used often enough, it will actually take up *less* physical space in the brain. This isn't because the pathway is weaker. It's because the pathway has become incredibly streamlined, and efficient, sort of like a flabby body that gets leaner as it grows stronger.

In Sally, this rule of brain change—neurons that fire together, wire together—has created a complex, strong pathway for habitual lying. When she told a lie, she felt thrilled, like a kid on a roller coaster. Also, her boyfriend would become more understanding and sympathetic in response to the lie, and Sally felt comforted. All these feelings were recruited into a neural pathway that also became linked to lying. (More about neurons and dopamine, the feel-good neurotransmitter, in a moment.) Sally's brain was like a pianist's, except that instead of recruiting neurons into the pathways for her hand, it was the pathways for lying, excitement, love, and comfort that had become so rich and interconnected.

I wanted Sally's brain to change which neurons were wiring together and firing together. This would be a little like asking a pianist to become a lacrosse player; in effect, Sally would learn to let one set of pathways wither while building up a completely different set.

Brain Change Rule Number 3: Repetition, Repetition, Dopamine

Almost twenty years ago, I attended the first conference on the neurobiology of post-traumatic stress disorder (PTSD), held in New York. I was on a steep learning curve regarding issues of trauma and abuse and was thrilled to hear many of the leading researchers in the field present their piece of the neurobiological puzzle. The results were fascinating. People suffering from post-traumatic stress disorder were found to have a dysregulated hypothalamic-pituitary-adrenal axis, too much amygdala activation, too much norepinephrine stimulation, and not enough cortisol production. I'll spare you the rest of the terminology, but suffice it to say that the sum total of these alterations in brain chemistry is a very reactive, irritable person.

We all wanted to help people with PTSD, but at the time, treatments for the disorder were poorly understood and difficult to implement. One research group stuck out, however, because their treatment was working. Edna Foa, a clinician and researcher from the University of Pennsylvania, was getting better than usual results in a group treatment designed for women who had a history of abuse, even when compared to other therapists who were using group treatments. Conference attendees were puzzled by the results. At one point, someone mentioned that Edna was an "unusual woman"—apparently this was code for a warm relational style that was very different from the standard detached application of treatment protocols. But no one (including me) went as far as to say that the relationships she was forming with clients or that the patients formed with one another in group therapy may have been a factor both in the research and in the success of her standardized treatment.

I can look back now and see that in Edna's program, the therapeutic and group relationship was likely a direct contributor to her success. The chemistry of healthy relationships enhances your ability to change your old patterns. Change is a form of new learning, and learning, at the microscopic level, is about making new neurons. We're making new synaptic connections, too: when we learn, axons and dendrites are reaching out to different neurons. The structure of the brain is being altered.

It's almost impossible for this neurological change to take place when you're feeling cut off from others. Isolation is a stressful state for both your body and brain, especially when you sense that you're being rejected or judged; your body reads it as a dangerous situation. It prepares you to answer the question, "How am I going to survive the next few hours?" As the sympathetic nervous system shifts into high gear, adrenaline races through your body, diverting energy to the large muscles in your arms and legs and helping your heart and lungs provide the oxygen that will fuel your body's fight-or-flight response. At these times, your body doesn't have the interest in or energy for building new synaptic connections for learning. It's simply busy saving itself.

When you are in healthy connection, your physiology is soothed, and you have a higher capacity for learning. Although you need a small amount of "good stress" to arouse your nervous system and give you a little boost of energy (think of how a skilled coach can put just enough pressure on you—but not too much—to help you play at your highest level), you can't effectively grow new synaptic connections unless you feel basically safe. Healthy relationships release a full cascade of chemicals that ease the way for learning. These include serotonin, which in certain areas of the brain has a calming effect, and norepinephrine, which has a focusing effect in small quantities. Oxytocin in particular appears to propel both relationships and learning. When you're in love or when you become a new parent, oxytocin floods the body; in a literal sense, it makes you want to reach out to another person, to hold and touch them. In his book *The Brain That Changes Itself,* psychiatrist Norman Doidge describes the theory that oxytocin encourages brain change by melting away some existing brain pathways so that you have room for new ones.[2] Again, this comes back to relationships—it allows us to change our old ways so that we can prepare for a different kind of life, one with a new partner or child. Oxytocin is released, although in smaller quantities, by friendships and other warm connections. If you want your brain to build a new pathway, you can speed along the process by enlisting oxytocin.

The neurochemical with the strongest capacity to encourage brain change may be dopamine, which is also released by growth-fostering relationships. I've already mentioned the dopamine reward system, which is so compelling that it creates addictions when dopamine pathways are connected to the wrong activities. By supplying your brain with a hit of dopamine from healthy relationships, you create a powerful connection between the activity you want to encourage and the body's natural cravings. You're offering the brain a reward for reshaping itself. Neuroscientist Martha Burns tells teachers to think of dopamine as the brain's "Save button," because when dopamine is paired with learning, the neural pathways associated with that new information are solidified and retained.[3]

For all these reasons, a healthy human relationship can be

the biggest asset you have when you are trying to change. At the same time, a healthy relationship without repetitive stimulation of a new pathway may not be able to effectively compete for brain space with existing unwanted neural pathways and their troublesome behaviors. This is why a third rule for brain change, whether you are in therapy or trying to change without professional support, is clear: repetition, repetition, dopamine.

Putting the Three Rules into Action

A visual may help illustrate how to put the three rules of brain change to work. One of our recent winters in New England was a bear, with more snowstorms than I can remember since my childhood in Maine. During the third major snowstorm in a single week, my friend's car became stuck at the end of our driveway, the back two wheels spinning helplessly on a patch of ice. Each time she stepped on the gas pedal, my friend's wheels spun faster and faster. The pathway transformed from a slick of ice atop the snow's surface to a deepening icy groove. The more she revved the engine, the deeper the car went, and the more stuck it became. This is what happens with habits and relational patterns. They may start as a small nuisance, but as the action is repeated over and over again, the neural pathway bulks up. The habit becomes entrenched.

When my friend's car was stuck, she needed a new pathway. The tires needed to land on a different section of the driveway that was not on the patch of ice. To free the car, I created a different pathway by packing salt and sand down into the deep groove. The wheels found some traction on this new surface. The car lurched onto the clean side of the driveway, and she was able to drive away.

Changing your brain and your old habits requires a similar shift, away from a neural pathway that is undermining your health to a more desirable pathway that stimulates both dopamine (to help solidify new habits) and healthy interpersonal connection (to stimulate the connected brain, decreasing stress and isolation and improving learning). Some people like to imagine that they are setting physical roadblocks down on the unwanted neural pathway, to block the impulse from traveling through. Other people like to imagine that they are lifting up the impulse that is originating in their brain and redirecting it to another pathway, one that's more pleasant. These images are an oversimplification of what happens in the brain, but this is an instance when simplicity has an advantage. When you feel yourself careening off into a bad habit, you might find that the habit's pull is so forceful that it's hard to remember what you need to do to change. But if you have a strong, clear image in mind, you are more likely to coax your mind into behaving differently.

Let's go back to Sally, who needed to decide on roadblocks she might set up to divert her from lying to her boyfriend.

There was no right or wrong answer, I explained. The first roadblock could be whatever allowed her to pause, for even a second, when she felt the temptation to lie. I encouraged her to be unafraid of taking very small steps, which are less overwhelming and easier to make than sweeping changes.

I had another recommendation to make. Many people come to define themselves by their bad habits or their failures; being able to recognize the bad habit as something apart from themselves is an important first step and can serve as a roadblock. Sally was able to set up a small roadblock on her lying pathway simply by recognizing the desire to lie as a way to change her physiology and make her feel better in the relationship. Her lies and the resulting knot of relational difficulties did not have to define her. Other people have set up similar roadblocks by saying things to themselves like "that's just my crazy thinking" or "this is just my body telling me that it's craving dopamine."

When she paused and labeled the urge to lie as simply a bad habit and an ineffective way to feel closer in a romantic relationship, Sally was able to remember that she was more than the habit that had frustrated her for years. This left her the mental flexibility to call up other, more important images of herself as a successful professional, a culturally sophisticated adult, and a caring person. These were positive, rich relational images of good connections. By changing her focus, Sally literally changed the stimulation to her brain. The pause also allowed Sally to gradually recognize that the impulse to lie wasn't really an impulse. It actually began much more gradually, when she was feeling lonely and starting to look forward to being with her boyfriend and feeling special, cared for. Her old relational templates did not allow her to linger in this state of positive anticipation, however. Almost immediately, she was flung into an intense fear of abandonment—a fear that her boyfriend wouldn't like her if he knew how she felt. This fear inevitably led to a lie designed to keep him sympathetic and interested. Sally began to label those thoughts as a part of her habit and could see how these thoughts had been recruited into the lying pathway she now wanted to starve.

As she got better at identifying the thoughts that preceded the lying, she worked on picking her mind up and off its groove—and then moving it to a more positive neural pathway. When she was alone and craving connection, she'd try imagining a time when she'd felt authentically connected with her boyfriend. If this didn't work, she might call him and say honestly that she missed him or that she felt low. Over time, she was also able to describe some of her lying behavior to a friend; they agreed that if Sally felt like lying, she would text the friend and tell her about it. One day Sally found herself conjuring up an old memory of a high school boyfriend who had adored her, no lying necessary. Each of these activities served as roadblocks *and* exercised healthier relational pathways. Although these pathways were withered from disuse, they were like desert plants that lie dormant but come back to life when they are given just a little water. When she engaged in these more positive actions, she felt the jolt of pleasure, the surge of dopamine.

Sally was not able to hold on to a positive image or activity every time she had the urge to lie, especially at the beginning of her attempt to change. Sometimes she ended up telling her boyfriend about how her grandmother had died, or how she had been mugged during her last trip abroad (all lies, including the trip). But as she practiced the skills for more honest relationships, this pathway strengthened, and it became easier to reroute her thoughts in its direction.

I want to stress that Sally had a long path ahead of her. It is not easy to change a very old habit, especially when you have as little experience with healthy relationships as Sally did. But it is definitely possible, especially if you have at least one safe relationship that will support you and your work. Unsurprisingly, Sally eventually broke up with her old boyfriend. I was worried when, within just a few weeks, she began dating someone new. Early in the relationship, a warning sign flashed. Sally moved into a new apartment, and he brought her a housewarming gift: a bottle of his favorite barbeque sauce to keep in her refrigerator. Sally and I talked about how confusing it was to receive a "gift" that was about him, not *her*. The next week, she explained to her new boyfriend that she appreciated the gift, but that she didn't like barbeque sauce herself. We cheered this small success— because, actually, it wasn't small. It was one of the first times she'd ever risked being honest this early in a relationship. To her surprise, her boyfriend did not mind that she had different tastes in condiments. Sally expressed her amazement to her friend, who had grown closer to her, and the friend reinforced the idea that a healthy relationship can tolerate different opinions and ideas. The combination of this safe friendship, along with regularly *not* lying, were literally rewiring Sally's brain for honest connection.

The takeaway message from this section of the book? Your brain can change, and most important for our purposes, your brain can change its patterns of relating to people. You can teach your new brain to be Calmer, more Accepting, more Resonant, and more Energetic—to bolster all four pathways that relate to growth-fostering relationships. That work begins with the book's next section: the C.A.R.E. program.

Chapter 4

THE C.A.R.E.
RELATIONAL ASSESSMENT

U p until now, we've talked about the underpinnings of relational neuroscience. Now it's time to launch that knowledge into practical use. This half of the book is about how to use the C.A.R.E. plan so that both your brain and your relationships are healthier.

Remember, the C.A.R.E. program consists of four parts. Each part represents a neural pathway for connection, and each of those pathways represents an aspect of relationships. When those pathways are up and running smoothly, you feel:

- **C**alm (via the smart vagus nerve)
- **A**ccepted (thanks to the dorsal anterior cingulate cortex)

- **R**esonant (mirroring system)
- **E**nergetic (dopamine reward pathway)

The four chapters that follow are full of suggestions and exercises for strengthening each pathway. You'll get the most benefit if you follow the entire program, but I often mix up the order of the steps to reflect a client's needs. You can do the same. A few people find that they need to focus on just one or two neural pathways instead of all four, and that's fine, too.

However, *everyone* needs to begin with the C.A.R.E. relational assessment, a tool you'll find in this chapter. Performing this assessment is like putting on 3-D glasses at the movies: it helps you see your relationships and your mind in a fuller dimension. I guarantee you'll have at least one aha moment in this chapter. Most people have more than one.

The C.A.R.E. relational assessment helps you discover:
- which of your relationships are most actively shaping your brain;
- what kind of neurological shaping is taking place inside you;
- relational patterns that may have been invisible until now;
- how to engage the C.A.R.E. plan so that you can get right to work on the neural pathways that need the most healing.

As you work on the assessment, expect insight. Expect a little discomfort; that's normal whenever you take time for honest reflection. Most of all, expect to finish this chapter with a plan for a more connected, more satisfying set of relationships. The work begins right here.

If You Skipped the Science Chapters . . .

You're fine. I happen to love the science behind relationships, but if that's just not your thing, you can begin here. Inside this chapter you'll find everything you need to know to get going, including bite-sized summaries of the four neural pathways that form the foundation for the C.A.R.E. plan.

How to Perform Your Relational Assessment

Do this exercise when you have about fifteen to twenty minutes of uninterrupted quiet time. It involves these five steps, which I'll describe in more detail on the following pages:

Step One: Identify your brain-shaping relationships
Step Two: Complete the C.A.R.E. Relational
    Assessment Chart
Step Three: Sort your relationships into safety groups

Step Four: Evaluate your C.A.R.E. pathways

Step Five: Optimize the C.A.R.E. program

Step One: Identify Your Brain-Shaping Relationships

Relationships shape your neural pathways, so let's figure out which ones are doing most of the relational shaping inside your brain. Later, you'll see *how* they are shaping it.

When I began using relational assessments, I would tell people to perform the assessment based on the most important relationships in their lives. Then I realized that when we think of the people who are most important to us, it's instinct to pick out just one or two of the highest-quality relationships. Yet those relationships aren't necessarily the ones that have the most effect on us. In reality, most people have a much wider network of acquaintances who leave a mark on their relational templates. And the more time you spend with someone—no matter whether the relationship is good, bad, strained, or workaday—the more it shapes your brain.

To get a more complete idea of the relationships that affect you, make a list of the adults you spend the most time with. By "time," I mean two things. One is *face time*: the people you see most often during the week. These can include friends and family, but don't be surprised if the names that pop up are people you may not feel all that close to: coworkers, neighbors, carpool partners, parents of your kids' friends, and the acquaintances you're always running into at the hardware store. I also want you to list the people who take up your *mental time.* These are the people who, for good or bad, are under your skin. You spend time thinking about them, worrying about them, writing loving e-mails to them, or feeling annoyed with them. Don't make the mistake of writing down only the names of the people you like the best!

Everyone is different when it comes to relationships, so don't worry about how many people are on your list. For instance, I am a person with many acquaintances but only a few very close friends. Some would call me an introvert. When I did this exercise, my list had seven people on it. In contrast, my best friend could easily jot down more names than I have items on my weekly grocery list. He has so many people in his world that a really complete list would take multiple sheets of paper. He is an extrovert for sure.

Now put those names in order of how much total time— whether it's face time or mental time—you spend with that person. The person you spend the most time with should be at the top of the list; the person you have the least contact with should be at the bottom. Put stars by the first five people on the list. These are the relationships that most dramatically influence your brain.

This exercise is already pretty interesting, isn't it?

Turn to the relational assessment chart on page 96. Now take the five starred names and, going from the first to the fifth, write in the name of each person across the top of the chart in the spaces provided.

A note: people who have been traumatized in their relationships often equate human interaction with pain. They may be so terrified of other people—or so turned off by them—that they see no alternative to their isolation. If this sounds like you and you are not able to think of any current relationships, think about relationships in the past that have been important to you, or about a pet that you have been able to love and trust. Remember, one goal of this program is for you to learn skills that will gently and safely expand your relational world. As long as you have a brain, you can change and connect.

Why Aren't Children on the Relational Assessment Chart?

Relationships with children are important. But healthy adults don't depend on children for their emotional needs, so kids don't appear on the relational chart. If you spend most of your time with children, you need to be sure that you have time and contact with supportive adults. This is doubly true for parents who are in a difficult relationship with a child—for example, a teen going through a turbulent adolescence—because the stress can and will impact your brain.

Step Two: Complete the C.A.R.E. Relational Assessment Chart

The C.A.R.E. Relational Assessment Chart makes twenty statements about relationships. For each of the five relationships you've written across the top, evaluate how frequently each of these statements is true, using this 1-to-5 scale:

1 = none or never
2 = rarely or minimal
3 = some of the time
4 = more often than not; medium high
5 = usually; very high

Try not to overthink this process; go with your gut. If you are struggling to come up with an accurate response to some of the statements, you can "try on" the relationship. Here's how: recall a recent interaction with the person, or create a mental image of a typical exchange between the two of you. Pay attention not just to the narrative that emerges in your mind but also to the feelings that arise in your body. Each relationship is coded within you as a complex mind/body image; that's why you have to listen to your body (in some cases, this is your gut in a literal sense) as well as to your brain when you are deciding how to rank each statement.

The C.A.R.E. Relational Assessment Chart

Answer the questions on a 1-to-5 scale: 1=None or never 2=Rarely or minimal 3=Some of the time 4=More often than not; medium high 5=Usually; very high	#1	#2	#3	#4	#5	Total Statement Score	C.A.R.E. Code
1. I trust this person with my feelings.							Calm
2. This person trusts me with his feelings.							Calm
3. I feel safe being in conflict with this person.							Calm
4. This person treats me with respect.							Calm
5. In this relationship, I feel calm.							Calm Accepted
6. I can count on this person to help me out in an emergency.							Calm Accepted
7. In this relationship, it's safe to acknowledge our differences.							Calm Accepted
8. When I am with this person, I feel a sense of belonging.							Accepted
9. Despite our different roles, we treat each other as equals.							Accepted

Answer the questions on a 1-to-5 scale:	#1	#2	#3	#4	#5	Total Statement Score	C.A.R.E. Code
10. I feel valued in this relationship.							Accepted
11. There is give and take in this relationship.							Accepted
12. This person is able to sense how I feel.							Resonant
13. I am able to sense how this person feels.							Resonant
14. With this person I have more clarity about who I am.							Resonant
15. I feel that we "get" each other.							Resonant
16. I am able to see that my feelings impact this person.							Resonant
17. This relationship helps me be more productive in my life.							Energetic
18. I enjoy the time I spend with this person.							Energetic
19. Laughter is a part of this relationship.							Energetic
20. In this relationship, I feel more energetic.							Energetic
Safety Group Score							

In a moment, I'll give you some tools for analyzing the chart. Most people, though, find that they have some immediate reactions, even before they do any kind of analysis. Take a minute to think about your own reactions now. Do you notice any patterns? Surprises?

The chart is a representation of the relationships that literally shape your brain. Remember the second rule of brain change:

Neurons that fire together, wire together.

This means that the more time you spend in a relationship, regardless of whether it is mutual or abusive, the more that relationship is actively shaping your central nervous system. Do you spend lots of time in relationships that you ranked with ones and twos? Your brain may be shifting to a state of chronic disconnection to protect you from the pain. On the other hand, if you spend most of your time in relationships marked by fours and fives, then your connected brain—your smart vagus nerve, your dorsal anterior cingulate cortex, your mirroring system, and your dopamine reward pathway—is being programmed to expect healthy relationships and to thrive in them. You are supporting your capacity to find joy and comfort in the context of the human community.

If your relationships score mostly in the low numbers, does this mean that you are bad at relationships? Absolutely not. Everyone spends some time in difficult relationships, and sometimes we are thrown into them through no choice of our own. Your challenge is to learn which relationships can be grown so that they are stronger and more supportive, and which ones you may eventually need to put aside. You'll also make it possible to create rewarding new relationships. Finally, you can learn how to inoculate yourself against very stressful relationships, such as those at work, that you may not be able to leave and cannot change.

At this point, don't write off any of your relationships unless you are clearly being abused. Instead, read on. You'll use the assessment to determine which steps of the C.A.R.E. program to use first. The C.A.R.E. program can help you lay down the neural circuitry that makes it easier to have growth-fostering relationships. Here's to a relational world ranked four and above.

Step Three: Sort Your Relationships into Safety Groups

As you go through the C.A.R.E. program, you'll perform exercises that are designed to improve your neural pathways for connection. You can do many of these on your own, but some of them ask you to practice new methods of interaction with another person. I promise that I won't ask you to try anything that feels too bizarre or too frightening; I firmly believe that baby steps are the best way to get where you want to go. But even when the steps are small, relationship changes make most of us feel uncomfortably vulnerable. Why? One reason is that most of us are wired to fear difference and change. Another is that our culture makes it really hard to be vulnerable; it doesn't teach the skills that can make relational change easier on everyone.

You can improve your chances of having a good experience with change if you take these small risks within relationships that are already fairly sturdy and flexible. Here, you'll sort your relationships into safety groups so that you can see which give you the room to try out new ways of relating.

Return to your relational assessment chart and add up the column of twenty numbers under each relationship. The maximum total score per relationship is 100 points (20 questions × high score of 5).

Using the following scale, sort your relationships according to these three safety groups:

HIGH SAFETY: 75 POINTS OR MORE

Relationships in this category are quite sturdy, with many 4s and 5s. A relationship in this group is a relatively safe place to try out new relational skills or to discuss concrete ways to support each other.

MODERATE SAFETY: 60–74 POINTS

These relationships are usually not the first place to turn when you need to express a difficult emotion or when you want to try out a relational skill that doesn't feel comfortable yet. Wait until you have more practice, and then you can try applying these skills to improve the relationship. In some cases, you may decide that you are willing to take the risk of letting the person know that you are open to making things better between the two of you. You may find that if the other person has more information about how to relate differently, he or she can meet you halfway.

LOW SAFETY: 0–59 POINTS

With their many 1s and 2s, relationships that are low in safety cannot tolerate much vulnerability or conflict. It's not wise to try new relational skills within this group, at least not right away, even if the people in this group are family members or longtime friends you feel you ought to be able to trust.

If a relationship is, frankly, abusive—emotionally, physically, or sexually—it is important for you to get help from an outside source (physician, therapist or counselor, religious leader, domestic violence specialist) to think of ways of extricating yourself from the relationship.

But some relationships in the low-safety category aren't abusive, just problematic. Often, bad relationships are bad because they are shaped by "power-over" dynamics, in which one person is dominant and the other is subordinate. You may be able to reset those dynamics, but this process will be much easier if you work on other, less risky relationships first.

Now that your safety groups are complete, do you see some of your relationships in a different way? If you need some time to absorb this new perspective, take it. Just remember that the goal of this exercise is not to search for the people who have done you wrong, and it's not to blame your parents for the ways they raised you. The goal is definitely not to make you feel bad about the current state of your relationships. So go ahead and note any discomfort you might be having, but come back. Even if all your relationships are low in safety, you'll learn more about how to improve your support system.

If you've made the rare discovery that each of your five relationships is in the safest group, please follow these instructions: put this book down, live your life, and call me. I could use some uncomplicated friends!

Step Four: Evaluate Your C.A.R.E. Pathways

Here, you'll use the assessment to gather information about your neural pathways for connection. Once you know more about your neural pathways, you'll have an entirely new understanding of your relationships. You'll see why some of them are rewarding and what makes others so difficult. Better still, you can use this information to customize the C.A.R.E. program to your needs. Most people who complete this step feel more positive about their innate ability to connect *and* the potential to make their relational network much stronger.

Remember, these are the four C.A.R.E. pathways:
Calm, promoted by the smart vagus nerve
Accepted, via the dorsal anterior cingulate cortex
Resonant, from the mirroring system
Energetic, from the dopamine reward pathways

Go back to the assessment chart that you've completed. For each of the twenty statements, add up the five numbers that appear across the row. Record that total under the heading "Total Statement Score." The maximum score for each statement is 25 (a maximum high score of 5 × 5 different relationships). These totals will help you identify the strength of the four major neural pathways for connection.

Calm: The Smart Vagus

The smart vagus is a nerve that transmits signals to decrease stress. It's also connected to your sense of relationships. Whenever you see a good friend, the smart vagus normally sends out soothing messages to your autonomic nervous system, telling your whole body to relax. But the smart vagus can get confused. You can be born with a genetic tendency to have poor vagal tone, meaning that it fails to send appropriate messages. Very stressful situations in childhood, or later in life, can also cause poor vagal tone. You may feel more threatened or anxious in social settings, and you may find it hard to trust people.

To assess the functioning of your smart vagus, add the total scores for all the statements whose C.A.R.E. Code includes the word "Calm." This includes statements one through seven. The maximum score for the smart vagus category is 175 (seven statements, each with a possible high scores of 25).

A Calm score of 135 to 175 indicates that you have good vagal tone. Your smart vagus is able to take in the messages from your primary relationships and translate them into calming, relaxing signals. You have relationships that help you manage the stress of everyday life.

If your Calm score is between 100 and 134, you feel stressed out and anxious more often than you'd like to. This tension may be the natural result of relationships that feel somewhat risky; these stimulate an appropriate response from your sympathetic nervous system. Or you may suffer from poor vagal tone, in which case you may currently have some good relationships—but your smart vagus can't send the stress-relieving messages that it's supposed to. You'll definitely want to investigate further, which you can do in the Calm part of the program.

A Calm score below 100 means that your relationships often feel unsafe; they frequently add to the stress in your life rather than diminish it. This could reflect significant problems in the quality of your current relationships. If those relationships are unsafe and unresponsive, you won't get the benefit of the smart vagus, and your stress-response system will be continually activated. A low score here could also be an indicator of a genetic tendency toward poor vagal tone or of past abusive relationships that blocked your smart vagus's ability to function. No matter what the cause, poor vagal tone leaves your nervous system reactive, always primed for the next attack. When a relationship feels chronically unsafe, it's often the case that neither your vagal tone nor your relationship is working well.

Accepted: The Dorsal Anterior Cingulate Cortex

The dorsal anterior cingulate cortex registers both physical and emotional pain. When you feel left out, it sends out a distress signal. Repeated experiences of feeling socially excluded can stress your dACC and lock it into a Fire position. When this happens, you feel all the pain of being socially excluded— even when people are trying to welcome you into their lives. To assess your dACC functioning, add the Total Statement Scores for lines five through eleven—these are all the statements with the C.A.R.E. Code that includes the word "Accepted." The maximum score is 175 (seven statements with a possible score of 25 each).

An Accepted score of 135 to 175 indicates that your dACC is well tuned. You tend to feel safe and unthreatened in your relationships, but when you are being excluded, your dACC sends a message of pain and distress. You benefit from a helpful signal that lets you know when to trust people and when something is wrong.

If your Accepted score is between 100 and 134, your emotional alarm system is somewhat reactive. You may often feel left out or as though you do not belong. Even when you spend time with others, you may have an underlying sense of loneliness. The Accepted part of the C.A.R.E. program can help you determine whether you are truly being left out and, if so, can help you take steps toward more supportive relationships. It can also tell you if a reactive dACC is sending you mistaken signals that leave you feeling unsafe and under attack even when people would like to be friendly with you. That same step can help you calm your dACC to give you more accurate feedback.

An Accepted score below 100 indicates that your relational alarm system is being chronically stimulated. This overactive system probably results from past or current destructive relationships—but it is also distorting the way you see *all* your relationships, even the ones that have the potential for warmth and mutual support.

Resonant: The Mirroring System

The mirroring system allows you to read other people's actions, intentions, and feelings with accuracy. When the mirroring system is working well, you feel a sense of resonance with others. When your mirroring system fails, you may feel that there's a wall between you and everyone else.

To assess the functioning of your mirroring system, add

the Total Statement Scores for lines twelve through sixteen. These are all the lines whose C.A.R.E. Code says "Resonant." The maximum score is 125 (five questions, each with a possible high score of 25).

A Resonant score between 95 and 125 reveals that your mirroring system is functioning well. Your relationships feel emotionally easy; you and your friends don't have to spend a lot of time explaining yourselves to each other. You understand most other people, and you feel that the people close to you can "see" who you truly are.

A Resonant score between 70 and 94 shows that you sometimes find other people confusing. Occasionally, important people in your life don't seem to "get" you, and in turn, you misread people's intentions or reactions more often than you would like. The exercises in the Resonant portion of the C.A.R.E. program can help activate and clarify your mirroring system.

If your Resonant score is below 70, you probably think of other people as baffling. You may find yourself shaking your head in bewilderment at friends and colleagues, saying, "I just don't understand you!" Some people with low Resonant scores get into trouble because they are overly suspicious; others are guileless, naively assuming that everyone around them always has sterling intentions. And *you* are misunderstood as well: when you try to be kind, you get accused of being sneaky or invasive. Or maybe you give off signals of romantic interest that you'd never intended. You find feelings uncomfortable and overwhelming. If this sounds like you, go directly to the Resonant step of the program, where you can more fully assess the activity of your mirroring system. You'll also discover ways to make subtle distinctions among different kinds of feelings—both yours and other people's.

Energetic: The Dopamine Reward Pathways

Dopamine is the pleasure neurotransmitter. Ideally, your dopamine reward pathways are linked up with healthy relationships, so connecting with other people stimulates feelings of energy and motivation. But when your relational world leaves you drained, paralyzed, and unhappy, you may find yourself seeking dopamine from other sources. You get your dopamine hits from food, alcohol, drugs, meaningless sex, or other addictive behaviors. One way to tackle bad habits and addictions is to rewire your dopamine pathways so that you get pleasure from your best relationships instead of your worst vices.

To determine your Energetic score, add the Total Statement Scores for statements 17 through 20. These are the statements whose C.A.R.E. Code is "Energetic." The total maximum Energetic score is 100 (four questions with 25 maximum points per question).

If your Energetic score is between 75 and 100, your dopamine pathways are plugged directly into relationships. You have good connections with other people, and those connections naturally supply you with more energy, more motivation, and more ability to act on behalf of yourself and your friends.

An Energetic score between 55 and 74 indicates that your relationships can sometimes feel unrewarding. You may have one or two relationships that you are truly enthusiastic about, but the others leave you feeling neutral and not so jazzed up. It's a good bet that you often turn to food, alcohol, or another source of dopamine as your consolation prize. Practicing the exercises in the program's Energetic step will help you redirect dopamine stimulation away from addictions (including "soft" ones, such as eating and shopping) and back toward healthy connections, significantly brightening your life.

A dopamine score of 54 or below reveals that the relationships in your life are draining. You may long for at least one close friendship, but you would rather be alone than participate in relationships that are unrewarding. You may rely on addictive, repetitive behaviors, such as substances or shopping, to give yourself a lift.

Step Five: Optimize the C.A.R.E. Program

You've got your chart, your scores, and your results. Now what? Be honest about where you're weak and where you're strong. Then decide how you'll work the steps of the C.A.R.E. program. Will you do them in order, or switch them around? Do all the steps, or select just a few?

I'm going to show you how three of my clients used their results for a clearer understanding of their relationships and to customize their C.A.R.E. program.

Jennifer: From Despair to Clarity

One of the most powerful benefits of the relational assessment is that it helps you put a name on what's bothering you. Then you can take concrete steps toward solutions.

This is exactly what happened to Jennifer, who called me for an appointment after a devastating week. She and her on-again-off-again boyfriend, Jakob, had an explosive fight after Jennifer playfully criticized the suit he wore to a friend's wedding. At the same time, Jennifer's sister, Claire, was giving her the silent treatment. Although Jennifer recognized this as a ploy often used within the family to punish certain behaviors, Jennifer was not sure what she had done to make her sister mad. Fearing that she simply "sucked" at relationships, she turned to the only place she knew of for help: the Internet. She Googled the word "relationship" and the Jean Baker Miller Training Institute appeared.

One week later, Jennifer was sitting nervously in my office, friendly and polite but making little eye contact with me. She described the fight with Jakob and explained that the two of them had repaired the rift in their usual way: a few days after the fight, Jakob texted Jennifer and called her a judgmental snob. Jennifer, feeling she deserved it, simply took the hit. They moved on quickly from there, making plans to go out with a small group of friends Friday night. They were talking again, but the interaction did little to deepen the trust between the two of them.

Jennifer predicted that the tension with her sister would be resolved in a similarly unsatisfying way. It had been a week since Claire's silent treatment had begun, and, Jennifer told me, she expected it to last exactly one week longer. The punishment for almost any infraction in her family, from speaking too bluntly to breaking a piece of heirloom china, was two weeks of being quietly shunned by the offended party. When the two-week period was over, the coldness thawed, and the relationship resumed as if nothing had happened.

Jennifer unflinchingly and, I thought, honestly offered detail after detail of her relational life, but she was frustrated that she couldn't assemble these details into a coherent picture. With no better way to understand her relationship problems, she fell back on the simple but depressing idea that she was bad with people.

At this point, I invited Jennifer to complete a relational assessment, explaining that labeling herself with the shorthand "bad with people" wasn't going to get her very far toward her goal of feeling better. I wanted both of us to have a clearer sense of the relationships that were currently shaping her brain and body.

Jennifer was drawn to this exercise. Her mind was naturally analytic—in fact, she was often accused of overthinking things by those closest to her—and she liked the idea of bringing more precision to her thoughts. She began by making a list of the people she saw during a typical week. Her list included her mother and sister; Jim, a coworker who occupied the cubicle next to hers; her boss, Frank; and her sort-of boyfriend, Jakob.

I asked Jennifer to sit quietly and to visualize a few interactions with each of these people, and to pay close attention to what she felt. Then she completed the assessment.

JENNIFER'S SAFETY GROUPS

High Safety: No one
Moderate Safety: Jakob and Claire
Low Safety: Mom, Jim, Frank

Jennifer's first response to seeing her relational safety groups was to say, "This proves I suck at relationships!"

I countered with an important truth: no one person "sucks" at relationships. Bad relationships are always formed by at least two people. You cannot be in a bad relationship alone! We agreed to replace her self-deprecating statements with one that was more accurate: the relationships that dominated Jennifer's life were disappointingly nonmutual.

From there, we took a closer look at Jennifer's relational safety groups. With two of her relationships in the moderate category and three posing a high risk, it was obvious that she had no safe, mutual relationships. This was not a shock to Jennifer. She had already told me that she really didn't trust

Jennifer's C.A.R.E. Relational Assessment Chart

Answer the questions on a 1-to-5 scale: 1=None or never 2=Rarely or minimal 3=Some of the time 4=More often than not; medium high 5=Usually; very high	#1 Jim	#2 Frank	#3 Claire	#4 Jakob	#5 Mom	Total Statement Score	C.A.R.E. Code
1. I trust this person with my feelings.	1	1	2	3	2	9	Calm
2. This person trusts me with his feelings.	2	1	3	4	3	13	Calm
3. I feel safe being in conflict with this person.	2	1	2	2	2	9	Calm
4. This person treats me with respect.	3	1	3	3	2	12	Calm
5. In this relationship, I feel calm.	2	1	3	4	3	13	Calm Accepted
6. I can count on this person to help me out in an emergency.	2	1	3	3	3	12	Calm Accepted
7. In this relationship, it's safe to acknowledge our differences.	2	1	3	4	2	12	Calm Accepted
8. When I am with this person, I feel a sense of belonging.	2	1	3	3	3	12	Accepted
9. Despite our different roles, we treat each other as equals.	2	1	4	4	2	13	Accepted

Answer the questions on a 1-to-5 scale:	#1 Jim	#2 Frank	#3 Claire	#4 Jakob	#5 Mom	Total Statement Score	C.A.R.E. Code
10. I feel valued in this relationship.	2	1	4	4	3	14	Accepted
11. There is give and take in this relationship.	1	1	3	3	2	10	Accepted
12. This person is able to sense how I feel.	2	1	3	3	2	11	Resonant
13. I am able to sense how this person feels.	3	1	4	3	3	14	Resonant
14. With this person I have more clarity about who I am.	2	1	3	3	2	11	Resonant
15. I feel that we "get" each other.	2	1	3	4	2	12	Resonant
16. I am able to see that my feelings impact this person.	2	1	3	3	2	11	Resonant
17. This relationship helps me be more productive in my life.	2	1	3	3	2	11	Energetic
18. I enjoy the time I spend with this person.	2	1	4	4	3	14	Energetic
19. Laughter is a part of this relationship.	2	1	3	3	3	12	Energetic
20. In this relationship, I feel more energetic.	2	1	3	4	2	12	Energetic
Safety Group Score	40	20	62	67	48		

anyone and that if she was to be successful in life she would have to do it all on her own. But Jennifer did have a few surprises coming. She wouldn't have thought of her relationship with her mother as particularly low in safety. She loved her mother. But after some thought, she came up with a more complex portrayal of the relationship. She recognized that it felt close but also rigid, without much room for either of them to make a misstep.

The very low scores for Jim and Frank came almost as a relief. They explained the sense of dread Jennifer felt every morning as she got ready for work at a small software company. She had to physically harden herself for an environment with an unsmiling, critical boss who openly pitted workers against one another in what seemed like a sadistic attempt to increase productivity. As we looked at her overall score for Frank, it was clear to both of us that this work relationship was emotionally abusive. Her relationship with Jim was only a little better. Although Jim was not in a position of power over Jennifer, he was generally quiet and dismissive of her.

Even at this early stage of our work together, before she had even finished interpreting her relational assessment, Jennifer had a new way of describing at least one aspect of her troubles: her relational world at work was stimulating stress pathways in her brain and body. This explained why she felt a slight but constant agitated buzz in her body throughout the week. Up until now, Jennifer had thought this feeling was just another sign that she was odd or not meant for normal human interaction.

I asked Jennifer to imagine that the five people on her chart took up all her relational time and then to determine the percentage of time she spent with each person. This is a useful imaginative exercise that makes patterns and trends more obvious. Jennifer's percentages looked like this:

Person	Percentage of Relational Time
Jim	30
Frank	30
Claire	15
Jakob	15
Mom	10

This breakdown made it clear to Jennifer that she spent 70 percent of her time (with Jim, Frank, and her mother) in relationships that felt unsafe and, in one case, fairly abusive. Spending that kind of time in difficult relationships can bring the rest of your relational world down, because they can adjust your template of what "normal" looks like. You can forget what respect and warmth feel like. You can forget that you even *want* to be treated well.

From a relational standpoint, a job change would be ideal for Jennifer—the sooner, the better. But she felt that quitting her job would be a stupid move. She visibly deflated as she realized that she knew of no other companies that were hiring.

"Is there *anyone* at work you can relate to?" I asked. I explained that even if Jennifer couldn't leave Frank and Jim behind, she could dilute the impact of those bad relationships by reducing the percentage of time she spent in them.

Jennifer immediately shook her head, but then she paused. There was a new hire, Emily. They had met briefly the week before, and Jennifer had liked her energy. Her spirits lifted a little as she thought about asking Emily to lunch and seeing if they could form an informal support network. We also speculated about whether there was potential to improve things with Jim. Was he merely responding to the threatening office environment in the same way Jennifer had, by shutting down and retreating to his cubicle? Would he, like Jennifer, appreciate an opportunity for safe connection?

At this point Jim was still a question mark, but Jennifer decided she would spend a moment each day making contact, saying hello, and asking how he was doing—in a professional way, just to see if there was any softening of his demeanor.

Of all Jennifer's relationships, the ones with her sister and her boyfriend were clearly the most mutually supportive. As Jennifer reflected on these two relationships, she felt that she was most able to be herself with Jakob. This thought came as a revelation, because they'd never had a long stretch of dating without fighting. Yet she felt more comfortable around Jakob than she did with most other people. He seemed to trust her, and she liked that feeling. A cycle of fighting and then breaking up is often a sign that something is awry in a relationship. Jennifer, however, was surrounded by people who couldn't tolerate relational differences—when a problem occurred, they moved to disconnect from her. With Jakob, at least she had a relationship with some flexibility, in which both parties could disagree, move away, and then come back together to engage in relational repair. We decided that this relationship was the one that could most easily tolerate some stretching and growing. When the C.A.R.E. program identified exercises that could help Jennifer expand her relational skills, she'd practice them with Jakob.

Jennifer's C.A.R.E. Pathways
Calm: **80 (low)**
Accepted: **86 (low)**
Resonant: **59 (low)**
Energetic: **49 (low)**

When we looked at her C.A.R.E. neural pathway scores, it was clear that Jennifer needed major work in all areas. Having an abusive relationship in your life, like the one with her boss, Frank, leaves lasting imprints on your central nervous system. Those changes make it harder for you to trust and feel safe with others. As we talked about this, Jennifer was reminded of her grandfather. Although he died when Jennifer was five years old, she remembered that he was a difficult man, nasty and critical of everyone around him. Were there traces of this relational style that ran throughout her family life? It seemed possible that Jennifer's neural pathways had been influenced by challenging relationships from the very beginning, although this was a matter we'd investigate more fully at a later date.

All of Jennifer's neural pathways were taxed. Her Calm score likely signified a weak smart vagus nerve, one that was easily overrun by the sympathetic nervous system's stress response. Given her low Accepted score, her dACC alarm system was likely to be highly sensitive, contributing to that unpleasant "buzz" she carried in her body. And no doubt from her Resonant numbers, Jennifer's mirroring system had taken a series of blows from the frequent periods of silent treatment her family had used to control her behavior. This was clear from her low scores and from her ongoing difficulty in making eye contact, a classic strategy for preventing connection.

Of the four neural pathways, Jennifer's dopamine system was the hardest to read. Her overall score was low at 49, but her very low scores with the two men at work were throwing off the decent scores she had with her sister and Jakob. Despite the number, there was clear evidence that Jennifer could enjoy herself in some relationships. And she did not appear to rely heavily on external sources of dopamine. She had no addiction, not even a mild one, to alcohol, drugs, shopping, food, or the like.

Overall, Jennifer's relational map indicated that she would benefit most by doing the whole program. The exercises in each step would help soothe and strengthen her connection pathways; she would also get plenty of education about what a healthy relationship looks and feels like. I also wanted Jennifer to think about a long-term solution to her work problem. As Jennifer developed a taste for mutual relationships, and as she left behind her self-concept as a person doomed to isolation, I was hopeful that she'd find it easier to network her way into a new job. At the very least, perhaps she could protect herself from the worst of Frank's behavior.

Dottie: A Simple Solution to Work Stress

Dottie, a college professor and activist, was neither a wallflower nor a bully. Confident, composed, and witty, she was able to speak her mind in a variety of circumstances. Out of curiosity, she attended a workshop I was teaching, and when she took a look at the C.A.R.E. assessment, she thought: *Interesting, but why bother? I already know I have a strong support system.*

Dottie began the assessment anyway, quickly and easily jotting down the names of her live-in boyfriend, friends, family members, and close colleagues. But when I explained that the list should include anyone she spent a good deal of time with, her eyes widened. Her relational scales had just tipped significantly. Two of the people she saw most often were the two people who caused her the most grief. One of these people was Ken, the head of her academic department and a man she had to see on a daily basis. Throughout the years, their relationship had grown heavy with tension. Although they were mostly civil to each other, sometimes that tension broke through in faculty meetings or yearly evaluations. The other person Dottie added to her assessment was a senior colleague, Cynthia, who treated Dottie in a bossy, condescending way.

Dottie's C.A.R.E. Relational Assessment Chart

Answer the questions on a 1-to-5 scale: 1=None or never 2=Rarely or minimal 3=Some of the time 4=More often than not; medium high 5=Usually; very high	#1 Luca	#2 Ken	#3 Cynthia	#4 Lisa	#5 Kim	Total Statement Score	C.A.R.E. Code
1. I trust this person with my feelings.	4	2	2	4	5	**17**	Calm
2. This person trusts me with his feelings.	4	2	2	4	5	**17**	Calm
3. I feel safe being in conflict with this person.	4	2	3	4	5	**18**	Calm
4. This person treats me with respect.	5	2	3	4	5	**19**	Calm
5. In this relationship, I feel calm.	5	2	2	4	4	**17**	Calm Accepted
6. I can count on this person to help me out in an emergency.	5	3	3	5	5	**21**	Calm Accepted
7. In this relationship, it's safe to acknowledge our differences.	5	3	3	4	5	**20**	Calm Accepted
8. When I am with this person, I feel a sense of belonging.	5	2	2	5	5	**19**	Accepted
9. Despite our different roles, we treat each other as equals.	5	2	3	4	5	**19**	Accepted

Answer the questions on a 1-to-5 scale:	#1 Luca	#2 Ken	#3 Cynthia	#4 Lisa	#5 Kim	Total Statement Score	C.A.R.E. Code
10. I feel valued in this relationship.	5	3	3	5	5	**21**	Accepted
11. There is give and take in this relationship.	5	2	2	4	5	**18**	Accepted
12. This person is able to sense how I feel.	4	2	2	4	4	**16**	Resonant
13. I am able to sense how this person feels.	4	2	3	5	4	**18**	Resonant
14. With this person I have more clarity about who I am.	5	3	1	4	5	**18**	Resonant
15. I feel that we "get" each other.	5	2	2	4	5	**18**	Resonant
16. I am able to see that my feelings impact this person.	4	2	2	4	5	**17**	Resonant
17. This relationship helps me be more productive in my life.	5	2	2	4	5	**18**	Energetic
18. I enjoy the time I spend with this person.	5	2	2	4	5	**18**	Energetic
19. Laughter is a part of this relationship.	5	2	2	5	5	**19**	Energetic
20. In this relationship, I feel more energetic.	5	2	2	5	5	**19**	Energetic
Safety Group Score	**94**	**44**	**46**	**86**	**97**		

DOTTIE'S SAFETY GROUPS

High Safety: Luca, Lisa, Kim
Moderate Safety: No one
Low Safety: Ken and Cynthia

Dottie's C.A.R.E. Pathways
Calm: **129 (moderate)**
Accepted: **135 (high)**
Resonant: **87 (moderate)**
Energetic: **74 (moderate)**

When we looked over her assessment, it was clear that Dottie's initial instinct had been correct: she did have a strong support system of largely mutual relationships. Although her scores for her C.A.R.E. pathways were in the middling range, it was obvious that the mostly high scores in her good relationships were pulled down by her two difficult colleagues. In a situation like this, it's tempting to say, "Oh, well, the numbers don't really reflect the reality. This lady has some annoying colleagues, but who doesn't? She's basically fine."

Not quite. Recall the first two rules of brain change:

1. Use it or lose it.
2. Neurons that wire together, fire together.

These tell us that the brain is influenced and sculpted by what it is most exposed to, and the relationships that were sculpting Dottie's brain on a daily basis were the ones that felt the least mutual, least safe, and most stressful. Instead of trying to work *with* Dottie, her colleagues Ken and Cynthia were constantly trying to establish power *over* her. Even with a lifetime of good relationships behind her, these two difficult relationships could powerfully affect Dottie's thinking and feelings. Although she had thick skin and didn't take her co-workers' power moves personally, Dottie felt distracted and extra tired when she had to "put up" with them. She was more likely to go home and isolate herself—and maybe eat a little more ice cream than was good for her—instead of spending her free time with her boyfriend or her friends. As we talked, Dottie realized that this isolation was making things worse: the percentage of relational time she spent with her difficult colleagues was increasing.

Unlike Jennifer, Dottie did not need to do a major over-haul of her relational world, but she did need to target the two relationships that had so much negative power. She drew up a two-step plan. Dottie knew that she couldn't change her relationship with her coworkers—she'd already tried—so she decided that they would occupy a lower ranking on the list of people she spent time with. She'd do this by increasing the time she spent in mutually supportive relationships; in es-sence, she'd move those good relationships up on the list. This was a pledge that was going to be difficult to honor. She thought of times when she'd been too busy to return friends' calls or hadn't followed through on plans to meet up. The thought of letting negative relationships shape her brain, however, was all the prompting she needed to put a few lunch dates on the calendar. She also realized that she was not using one of her most obvious sources of growth and support: her partner, Luca. After her long workdays, Dottie had been content to tuck away into her study at night, feeling the relief of not having to interact with anyone. By the time they went to bed, she and Luca had often not spoken more than a few sleepy sentences to each other. She explained to Luca what she'd learned from the seminar and they made an effort to spend more connected time together at the end of the day—not just venting their problems, but savoring each other's company. Finally, Dottie concluded that she could benefit from the strategies in the Calm step to help her get through the inevitable meetings with her challenging colleagues. She also decided to try a few ideas in the Energetic step to keep her from turning to sweets when she needed a dopamine boost after a hard day.

A couple of weeks after Dottie returned to work, she sent me a note. Her two-pronged plan was already helping: she was feeling more energetic and had noticed a reduction in her daily stress level.

Rufus: Addicted to Energy

Rufus saw himself as an ordinary guy with a big problem. He'd graduated the year before from a local community college and found a job within three months at a biotech company. He liked his job, but to him, a job was just a way to make money and pay his bills. It was not a passion and never would be. He was a guy who was comfortable living an anonymous life—again, this is how Rufus described himself to me—without major highs and lows, a guy who did not stir extreme reactions in anyone. He was part of the background, blending into the fabric of life. He looked forward to weekends and hanging out with some of his buddies, drinking a few beers and watching whatever game was on television. He dated occasionally, but no one had swept him off his feet.

Three years ago, when Rufus was eighteen, he discovered Internet porn. He was online looking over his next picks for his fantasy football team when a pop-up screen appeared in front of him featuring a provocative picture of a young woman. He wasn't sure why he clicked through. In retrospect, he thought he might have just been bored. What Rufus discovered going through this portal was a virtual world he never knew existed. He had heard his friends describe images they'd seen online, but he'd always assumed they were making up most of the details.

That night Rufus stayed up until four a.m. roaming from one porn site to another, each one giving him a little hit of energy. This was a new feeling for him, very different from his predictable, mellow life. He was not even sure he liked this feeling at first. It was unfamiliar and uncomfortable. But he returned to the site the next night, and the next.

Very quickly, Rufus was spending hours every night browsing for new and different porn sites. He shared this new world with no one and figured the only drawback was that he was getting less sleep at night. After three months of staying up late and dragging himself to work in the mornings, he realized he was hooked and tried to cut back, but was simply unable to. It was as if the websites had taken over his brain and body. Rufus came to my office when he found himself unable to resist sneaking peeks at work during lunch or whenever he felt bored. Before he was caught using his work computer for porn, he said, he wanted to get control of himself.

I explained that although we would clearly have to address the big problem of porn, addictions rarely happen in isolation. We'd use the C.A.R.E. assessment to create a more complete picture of his world. When I asked Rufus to come up with the five people he spent most of his time with, he quickly mentioned his card-playing buddies, Drew and Kevin. Rufus loved his mother and sister, Angela, and usually had some contact with them during the week, so they were listed. But after that it was slim pickings. I needed to prompt him about work relationships, and he did not seem to think of his colleagues as people with whom he had relationships. They were simply people at work. Then he came up with Wendy, who sat in the cubicle kitty-corner from his. Although Rufus was surrounded by coworkers, Wendy was the only one who made an impact on him. She often had a smile on her face and always asked how his latest project was coming along.

Although Rufus was nearly stumped by the task of coming up with five relationships, completing the questionnaire was easy for him. In fact, as Rufus went through the questions, his answers were unusually concrete. Most people worry a little over their answers and have the urge to fiddle with them, but Rufus didn't. I wondered whether he was unable to access his feelings well enough to form nuanced impressions of his relationships. Or perhaps he was merely decisive.

It was tempting to think of Rufus as a person who suffered from a straightforward case of addiction. Fix the addiction, problem solved. But the relational assessment showed us that unless Rufus attended to a few other areas, he'd have very little chance of beating his addiction in a permanent way.

RUFUS'S SAFETY GROUPS

High Safety: No one
Moderate Safety: No one
Low Safety: Drew, Kevin, Mom, Wendy, Angela

Given Rufus's self-definition as someone content to blend into life's scenery, doing his own thing, it was not surprising that his overall scores on his assessment show that he was deprived of growth-fostering relationships. There was little variation in how he scored each relationship (the scores stayed between 47 and 53, only a six-point difference), and each of them was in the lowest category of relational safety. This fit

Rufus's C.A.R.E. Relational Assessment Chart

Answer the questions on a 1-to-5 scale: 1=None or never 2=Rarely or minimal 3=Some of the time 4=More often than not; medium high 5=Usually; very high	#1 Drew	#2 Kevin	#3 Mom	#4 Wendy	#5 Angela	Total Statement Score	C.A.R.E. Code
1. I trust this person with my feelings.	2	2	2	2	2	**10**	Calm
2. This person trusts me with his feelings.	2	2	2	2	2	**10**	Calm
3. I feel safe being in conflict with this person.	3	2	2	2	2	**11**	Calm
4. This person treats me with respect.	3	2	3	4	3	**15**	Calm
5. In this relationship, I feel calm.	3	3	3	3	2	**14**	Calm Accepted
6. I can count on this person to help me out in an emergency.	3	2	4	4	4	**17**	Calm Accepted
7. In this relationship, it's safe to acknowledge our differences.	2	2	2	2	3	**11**	Calm Accepted
8. When I am with this person, I feel a sense of belonging.	3	3	4	2	4	**16**	Accepted
9. Despite our different roles, we treat each other as equals.	3	3	3	3	3	**15**	Accepted

Answer the questions on a 1-to-5 scale:	#1 Drew	#2 Kevin	#3 Mom	#4 Wendy	#5 Angela	Total Statement Score	C.A.R.E. Code
10. I feel valued in this relationship.	3	3	4	3	3	**16**	Accepted
11. There is give and take in this relationship.	2	2	3	3	2	**12**	Accepted
12. This person is able to sense how I feel.	2	2	3	2	3	**12**	Resonant
13. I am able to sense how this person feels.	2	2	3	2	3	**12**	Resonant
14. With this person I have more clarity about who I am.	2	2	2	2	2	**10**	Resonant
15. I feel that we "get" each other.	3	3	2	3	2	**13**	Resonant
16. I am able to see that my feelings impact this person.	2	2	2	2	2	**10**	Resonant
17. This relationship helps me be more productive in my life.	2	2	2	3	2	**11**	Energetic
18. I enjoy the time I spend with this person.	4	3	3	3	3	**16**	Energetic
19. Laughter is a part of this relationship.	3	3	2	3	2	**13**	Energetic
20. In this relationship, I feel more energetic.	3	2	2	2	2	**11**	Energetic
Safety Group Score	**52**	**47**	**53**	**52**	**51**		

with my sense that not only would Rufus have a hard time finding relationships to stretch in, but that he also had very little knowledge about how he might do this. The C.A.R.E. plan is *always* based on making small, unthreatening changes, but with Rufus, we'd have to be extra cautious in how we proceeded.

Rufus's C.A.R.E. Pathways
Calm: 88 (low)
Accepted: 101 (moderate)
Resonant: 57 (low)
Energetic: 51 (low)

There's a saying among physicians that the presenting problem—the problem that clients identify as their main issue—is never the *real* problem. That's not quite true. Porn addiction was definitely a real problem and a serious threat to Rufus's job and well-being. But although Rufus came in specifically for help with his addiction, it wasn't the whole story. He didn't have the exact words for it, but he seemed to want me to know about a curious flatness in his life. He claimed to like his routine, but he gave no sign that his life was satisfying. "Inert" was a better word. Porn gave him not just sexual gratification but a missing spark of energy. In fact, it was the hit of energy that brought him back to porn again and again. Until Rufus completed his assessment, this energy problem hovered in his peripheral vision, almost out of sight. When he looked at his numbers, he could see it clearly.

Remember, dopamine is what gives you good energy and motivation. When Rufus and I looked at his assessment, we saw that his Energetic score—which reveals the ability to get dopamine from relationships—was very low. No surprise there. Here's what was interesting: some people with low Energetic scores are in difficult, constantly frustrating relationships. Others have almost no relationships at all. That makes sense: bad relationships, or no relationships = low dopamine. But Rufus's relationships were actually okay. Not intimate or satisfying or truly safe, mind you, but okay. He liked hanging out with his buddies and his family. You'd think he would get at least a middling amount of energy from these contacts, but he was getting almost none. No wonder he didn't feel motivated to do any more at work or in life than he absolutely had to.

Was Rufus just a guy who didn't need people? No. Everyone is born with the capacity for getting dopamine from connections with people around them. Somewhere along the way, Rufus's dopamine system had become disconnected. His brain was like a toaster whose electrical cord had been unplugged from the socket. The socket can provide energy, but the signal can't travel down the cord to the toaster. The result: no toast. In Rufus's case, no mental energy, either.

The low Energetic score accounted for some of the flatness Rufus experienced, but not all of it. Look at the rest of his assessment. It describes a person who is not anxious or sad or irritable, which is a good sign. It also shows someone who does not have easy access to emotional information. For example, Rufus's Resonant score was also low, almost as low as his Energy. He had a hard time reading people or knowing when other people were accurately reading him. His Calm score, at 88, was also low; this was mostly due to the march of 2s across the statements about sharing feelings. At 101, his score for Accepted was in the moderate category (we celebrated this small victory), reflecting he felt safe and not overly stressed. He explained that he felt a definite sense of belonging with his mother and sister and that it never occurred to him that he might be ostracized with his friends or at work. I was glad that he was tight with his family; but in the rest of his relationships, he seemed to be missing something. Again, it wasn't that he had a bad feeling about his friends or colleagues; it was that he didn't have much of a feeling about them at all.

All in all, the relational flatness in Rufus's brain and body was a perfect setup for an addiction. Yes, he liked the porn itself, but he was really addicted to the feeling of finally having his dopamine system stimulated. As he said, he felt energized after viewing porn, in a way he'd never felt before.

Rufus needed a plan that would help him to do two things: reconnect his dopamine reward system to relationships (not porn), and develop more knowledge about how people interact. It was clear that Rufus would benefit from the entire program. But in his case, it made sense to rearrange the order of the steps.

ENERGETIC: Rufus's Energetic (dopamine) problem was the most urgent. He'd start with this step, which would help him disconnect his dopamine reward pathways from porn and reconnect them to healthy relationships.

RESONANT: By increasing the strength of his mirroring system, Rufus would make his connections to other people more satisfying. This would give him a larger supply of good feelings to send down the dopamine trail, resulting in more energy.

CALM: Although a low score here often results in anxiety or stress, Rufus seemed fairly placid. By increasing his vagal tone, he'd feel something richer than the blank dullness he was accustomed to. He'd feel content.

ACCEPTED: Rufus's dACC scores were decent, and he was not particularly concerned about having a sense of belonging. At this point, we decided not to focus on this step. I felt that as he developed a more textured sense of relationships, it was possible that he would begin to worry about inclusion or exclusion. If that happened, we could always go back and add this step.

We now had the outline of a plan. I didn't expect the plan to turn Rufus into Mr. Sensitivity, and I don't think he wanted the title. But I knew that if he could see life with a broader palette of relational colors, he would do more than end his addiction. He'd feel more animated and alive.

Ready to begin the C.A.R.E. program? The next step—strengthening the smart vagus to feel Calmer—begins on the next page.

Chapter 5

C IS FOR CALM

Make Your Smart Vagus Smarter

Signs that a relationship strengthens your Calm pathway:
I trust this person with my feelings.
This person trusts me with his feelings.
I feel safe being in conflict with this person.
This person treats me with respect.
In this relationship, I feel calm.
I can count on this person to help me out in an emergency.
In this relationship, it's safe to acknowledge our differences.

It feels terrible to be tense and irritable. Imagine what life was like for Juan, who felt tense and irritable *all the time*. On the Monday morning before I met Juan, he woke up feeling even worse than usual. He'd stayed up late watching football with a couple of friends the night before. They drank too much and ate too much, and his favorite team lost in overtime. The next morning, electric surges of rage shot through his body. He was angry about the game, and he was angry in general. Just the sound of toast crunching in his mouth threatened to push him over the edge. Juan considered calling in sick to his job as a computer programmer, but he was working on a new team project and the first meeting was scheduled for ten a.m. He showered and walked to the subway.

When he arrived at work, Juan could feel the tension building inside him. When he felt this way, the people around him seemed to become incredibly stupid. He didn't want to deal with their questions or hear stories about their weekends, so he sorted through his e-mail with earphones on, hoping no one would try to talk to him. But a new employee, Veronica, approached from behind and tapped him on the shoulder. He jolted from his chair, surprising them both. He sat down quickly and told her to leave him alone.

Juan hated meetings, particularly large team meetings intended to let everyone hear everyone else's thoughts about a new project. On a good day, Juan could barely sit through a meeting as people "threw out" their ideas. On a bad day, he rolled his eyes, snorted, or zoned out. In each of his evaluations at the company, Juan's boss praised him for his sharp analytic mind and computer skills but repeatedly told him he needed to change his attitude, his lack of interpersonal skills would prevent him from moving up. To Juan, this feedback felt like an attack, and another example of other people's annoying behavior.

Juan entered the meeting room ten minutes late, hoping to miss the opening chitchat. As his colleagues went around the table and described their thoughts about the project, Juan struggled to keep his patience. This felt like an unnecessary, self-indulgent step, aimed to please his touchy-feely boss. When Juan's turn came to "share," he gave a brief, monotone description of his role in the project, making eye contact with no one.

Midway through the meeting, Juan was asked how they might add new graphics to an existing demo product. His boss had told him that colleagues valued his skills; that's why they routinely turned to him with difficult problems. He enjoyed using his analytic mind to quickly break down even the most difficult problems and come up with plans that usually stunned his colleagues. But after Juan shared his ideas, a more junior member of the team spoke out, questioning the advice Juan had just given and suggesting an alternative approach. The electricity surged again, and Juan snapped. Furious, he stood up at the table and berated the young man. When Juan stopped yelling, the room was deathly quiet—until his boss asked him to leave the meeting. Juan stormed out of the room, slamming the door behind him. Later that morning his boss suggested Juan leave for the day and return to meet with him the next morning. Juan left the building, afraid he had gone too far this time and was likely to lose his job. But he didn't lose his job, as he found out the next day: he was referred to me for counseling.

. . .

When I met Juan, I was struck by his inability to sit still. Some part of his body was always in motion. For most of our meeting, his right leg bounced rhythmically. He picked at his fingers. He chewed gum, too—not a slow, relaxed chew but the kind of intense chewing you see in baseball players during a game. I could see the muscles of his jaw tighten over and over again. Despite this activity, Juan didn't look animated. He looked exhausted.

Juan knew that family members and coworkers described him as a hothead and that he reacted to many interpersonal exchanges with impatience. He appreciated that his job allowed him to spend hours interacting with his computer and not with people. He did occasionally have lunch with a colleague, but more often than not he ate at his desk, working comfortably between bites.

As we talked, Juan groaned and shook his head, looking at the floor.

"You groaned," I said. "What was that about?"

"I really don't want to be *that guy*," he said. "The Computer Guy with Anger Issues."

In truth, a lot of people suffer from jumpiness and irritability, and they work in all kinds of professions. Some are able to make it through the workday without exploding; these people often save up their tension for the unfortunate family members who wait for them at home. Some people aren't hostile at all, but they find interpersonal interactions so stressful that they want to jump into bed and pull up the covers after a trip to the grocery store. Some drink. A lot. (These are the people who need to "take the edge off.") I've always suspected that all these folks are underrepresented in therapy offices, in part because therapy sounds like fifty long minutes of irritating interaction, but also because they fear labels. *Something is terribly wrong with you,* they imagine me saying. *Here, let me show you this textbook that explains the word for people who can't handle being around others.*

But every person who's come to my office has been endlessly complex and interesting—and shorthand labels, even diagnoses, can never capture a soul's complexity. There's no judgment here: people with chronic interpersonal stress are usually relieved to know that their tension is not a character flaw or a personal failure. It's simply a problem with the Calm neural pathway. Specifically, this kind of constant relational stress is related to low tone in the smart vagus. Low vagal tone makes it hard to feel relaxed in the presence of others.

The autonomic nervous system contains three branches that help you react appropriately to threats: the sympathetic nervous system, which stimulates the fight-or-flight response when you are in danger; the parasympathetic nervous system, which brings on the freeze response when your life is threatened; and the smart vagus, which has the power to block the fight, flight, and freeze responses when you are feeling safe. At one end, the smart vagus feeds directly into the muscles of facial expression, vocalization, and swallowing, as well as the tiny muscles of your inner ear. At the other end, the smart vagus innervates the heart and lungs. When the smart vagus is working the way it should, it can "see" friendly expressions on the faces of people around you and "hear" warm voices. At these signals, the heart and lungs slow down into a relaxed pattern. In effect, the smart vagus has the power to tell the sympathetic and parasympathetic nervous systems: *I've surveyed the territory and things are okay. Your stress responses are not needed right now; it's safe to relax.* If the smart vagus doesn't get that input, it sends a different message: *The world looks pretty dangerous out there. Probably a good idea for you to mobilize, in case something bad goes down.*

I've mentioned that although the neural pathways for connection are constantly shaping themselves through your relationships, it's during childhood when these pathways are most malleable. The smart vagus needs stimulation from caring faces and voices in order to wire together with networks of nerves that associate that visual and audio input with safety. It needs to experience the relational qualities, like trust and the ability to feel safe during conflict, that strengthen the Calm pathway. Most important, the smart vagus—like a muscle—needs to be used to develop good tone. When that doesn't happen, the smart vagus doesn't grow strong, and it doesn't learn to associate relationships with serenity and safety. A person with low vagal tone may intellectually understand that he is surrounded by supportive, encouraging people and still feel terribly threatened *around those same people,* because his smart vagus isn't able to tell his stress-response systems to stand down. When vagal tone is very low, all relationships feel threatening.

Juan's smart vagus pathway was still under construction when, at age six, his mother died in a fiery car crash. His father, who was busy trying to keep his auto-body business afloat, had little time to nurture and care for his six children. Although Juan's sister, Blanca, tried to raise him, she was young herself—only twelve years old—when their mother died. And neither was able to protect themselves from their father, who yelled at them and sometimes hurt them. Instead of being exposed to soothing parental expressions, Juan became skilled at reading a different set of emotions. When his father came home with his eyes narrowed and his mouth pressed into a line, Juan knew to tread lightly and stay out of his father's way. When his father started yelling before even entering the house, Juan understood that it was time to take cover. On those nights, Juan wasn't sure he would live to see the morning. Juan's nervous system developed in a manner that was appropriate to this environment. His sympathetic nervous system was on almost all the time, its nerve pathways becoming muscular and efficient, while his smart vagus withered from disuse.

There was one reliable way Juan could relax and feel safe, and that was when he was alone. Studying computers was a godsend: the intricacies fascinated his detail-oriented brain, and there was little interpersonal interaction. When someone did approach him, even if just for a conversation, his body reacted with a surge of adrenaline, followed by anger or fear.

Early in life, he learned the route to staying safe and to minimizing those unsettling surges of stress: avoid people whenever possible.

As Juan became an adult, he had more control over the safety of his immediate world. But he still had an overprotective nervous system with a powerful fear response, and it was a significant barrier to healthy relationships. Nevertheless, Juan did have a social life. He still spent time with his family, even his father, and felt close to Blanca. He had a best friend, Bob, and they hung out with a small circle of friends. Juan dated quite a bit, though he'd had only one long-term relationship. That ended when his girlfriend decided she could no longer take Juan's reprimands and lectures.

You can see Juan's C.A.R.E. assessment on the following pages. Below, we'll look at how the different relational safety groups relate to the Calm pathway. We'll also see how Juan's safety groups shaped up.

Relational Safety Groups and the Calm Pathway

There are some patterns that tend to appear in people with weak Calm pathways, and some of these can be described within the three relational safety groups:

High safety (75–100 points): Low vagal tone means that it's hard for you to feel safe around other people. Given that Juan showed the classic signs of low vagal tone (irritability, anxiety, anger), it's not surprising that he had no relationships that helped him feel safe.

Moderate safety (60–74 points): If you have a weak Calm pathway, your closest relationships might be found here, in the moderately safe group. This may reflect a fear of trusting people, or it might mean that you don't have anyone in your life right now who is truly safe. I thought it was pretty good news, actually, that both Juan's sister, Blanca, and his friend Bob scored between 60 and 75 points, meaning that they felt at least somewhat safe to him. It was likely that as Juan learned skills to manage his overactive sympathetic nervous system, those relationships would improve. In turn, having safer and more rewarding relationships would help strengthen Juan's vagal tone.

Low safety (less than 60 points): Three of the relationships that took up major time and space in Juan's life scored below 60. These were relationships that were making his life worse, not better, because they exercised his sympathetic nervous system so frequently. Two of these people were from the office: his boss and a coworker. When they were around, Juan felt out of sync, as if everyone expected him to be as sociable as they were. This feeling of not quite measuring up could leave him irritated and then enraged. It didn't matter that when Juan described these guys to me, they actually sounded pretty friendly; his weak smart vagus kept him from feeling safe in these relationships. I didn't think Juan benefited from having his stress pathways constantly stimulated. But I wondered if, eventually, there would be potential for these work relationships to improve.

Juan's father was a different story. Juan's father had given

Juan's C.A.R.E. Relational Assessment Chart

Answer the questions on a 1-to-5 scale: 1=None or never 2=Rarely or minimal 3=Some of the time 4=More often than not; medium high 5=Usually; very high	#1 Blanca	#2 Dan (boss)	#3 Bob	#4 Sam (coworker)	#5 Father	Total Statement Score	C.A.R.E. Code
1. I trust this person with my feelings.	3	2	2	2	1	**10**	Calm
2. This person trusts me with his feelings.	2	2	2	2	2	**10**	Calm
3. I feel safe being in conflict with this person.	2	2	2	2	1	**9**	Calm
4. This person treats me with respect.	4	3	2	2	1	**12**	Calm
5. In this relationship, I feel calm.	3	2	2	2	1	**10**	Calm Accepted
6. I can count on this person to help me out in an emergency.	4	3	2	3	2	**14**	Calm Accepted
7. In this relationship, it's safe to acknowledge our differences.	3	3	3	2	2	**13**	Calm Accepted
8. When I am with this person, I feel a sense of belonging.	4	3	3	3	3	**16**	Accepted
9. Despite our different roles, we treat each other as equals.	3	4	4	3	2	**16**	Accepted

Answer the questions on a 1-to-5 scale:	#1 Blanca	#2 Dan (boss)	#3 Bob	#4 Sam (coworker)	#5 Father	Total Statement Score	C.A.R.E. Code
10. I feel valued in this relationship.	3	4	3	4	3	17	Accepted
11. There is give and take in this relationship.	3	3	3	3	2	14	Accepted
12. This person is able to sense how I feel.	5	3	3	2	2	15	Resonant
13. I am able to sense how this person feels.	3	2	3	2	3	13	Resonant
14. With this person I have more clarity about who I am.	4	3	3	2	1	13	Resonant
15. I feel that we "get" each other.	4	3	3	2	2	14	Resonant
16. I am able to see that my feelings impact this person.	3	4	3	3	2	15	Resonant
17. This relationship helps me be more productive in my life.	3	3	3	2	2	13	Energetic
18. I enjoy the time I spend with this person.	4	2	5	2	2	15	Energetic
19. Laughter is a part of this relationship.	4	2	5	2	2	15	Energetic
20. In this relationship, I feel more energetic.	3	2	4	2	2	13	Energetic
Safety Group Score	67	55	60	47	38		

up drinking years ago, but he was still a harsh and critical man. Though Juan was no longer an abused child, this relationship continued to weaken his Calm pathway and build up his sympathetic nervous system. This situation had to change.

Irritable . . . or Introverted?

Don't confuse irritability with introversion. Introversion is a normal, inborn personality trait. Introverts tend to be quieter and more reserved than extroverts. Being quiet and solitary is crucial for introverts, because it helps them feel refreshed. But introverts with healthy nervous systems definitely enjoy relationships. It's just that they prefer to be with a few close friends rather than go out with a big group of casual friends to a loud party. Their intimate friendships give their C.A.R.E. pathways plenty of stimulation and help them stay in good relational shape.

Introverts may be sensitive, and they're not at their best during large gatherings. But as a general rule, person-to-person interactions aren't likely to make them anxious and angry. They aren't exhausted by having to talk to a cashier at the convenience store. They can listen to a coworker's request without blowing a fuse. Whether you're an introvert or an outgoing extrovert, feeling irritable, anxious, and angry in your relationships is a sign that something is wrong—possibly that you're suffering from poor vagal tone.

Understanding Your Own Calm Score

Add up your scores for the statements whose C.A.R.E. Code includes the word "Calm." (That's statements 1 through 7.) Here's what the total number tells you:

When your C score is between 135 and 175: You've got healthy vagal tone, which means your Calm pathway is strong. Your smart vagus is robust and networked into neural pathways that can recall plenty of calming faces and voices; it's experienced at detecting when new people are friendly and when they're not. When you're around supportive people, your smart vagus transmits a calming message to your sympathetic and parasympathetic nervous systems. Being around your close friends helps you wind down and relax.

When your Calm score is between 100 and 134: Your close relationships don't always help you feel relaxed and comfortable. There can be a few reasons for this. One is that the people you spend most of your time with aren't trustworthy. The other is that your smart vagus isn't as strong as it could be, which means that even when you're with people you trust, your brain doesn't get the message to relax. Actually, both these reasons could come into play, because when you spend lots of time with people you can't trust, your smart vagus doesn't get exercised as frequently. As a result, your vagal tone gets weaker. A look at your relational safety groups can help you figure out whether you're spending too much time in low-safety relationships.

When your Calm score is lower than 100: Any Calm score below 100 is a low number. This is where Juan's score fell. The scores for all four of Juan's pathways were on the low side, but at 78, his Calm score stuck out. Given his chronic irritability and abusive upbringing, this was not a surprise. It wouldn't have made sense for his smart vagus to have good tone, because his smart vagus pathway was shaping itself at a time when his world was the opposite of safe and trustworthy. A very low Calm score usually describes a person who feels hyperalert and jumpy around people, and that fit my impression of Juan.

A low Calm score is a bad news/good news situation. Of course it's bad news that it's so hard to be around people— but you probably already know that you've been suffering. The good news is that a few therapies can help you feel a lot better, quickly.

Most people with low Calm scores have very few relationships that feel safe. Some have no safe relationships at all. There may be people on your list who are emotionally abusive (like Juan's father) or physically dangerous. There may also be others who are quite decent—it's just that you may be unable to pick up the messages of safety that their expressions and words are sending. As your reactive stress responses settles down, some of those relationships may feel more rewarding.

Strengthen Your Calm Pathway:
Ways to Feel Calmer and Less Stressed

For everyone with a weak Calm pathway, the first step in feeling better is education. Juan in particular was not used to thinking about his feelings and reactions to the world. When I asked him about friends and romantic relationships, he shrugged the question off by saying the words I hear so often: "I'm not good at relationships." He, like so many other people, believed he had been born like this.

Of course, he hadn't been born "like this"—he was born with the reflexes to connect with people, but he needed healthier relationships to build flourishing neural pathways for connection. Using a computer metaphor, I talked with him about the neural pathways for connection that are downloaded into each of us at birth. He was interested in this idea and became engaged in the neuroscience—a very good sign. We talked about how his nervous system had been formed in an environment of both traumatic loss (his mother's death) and constant threat (his father's emotional and physical violence). His neural pathways for healthy connection had not been stimulated enough to grow well. It was clear to both of us that until we could turn the volume down on his overactive sympathetic nervous system, he could not move out of the deep isolation he felt. In a self-protective move born out of experience, his brain was telling him to be angry and scared.

For anyone struggling with chronic irritability and

anxiety, learning to feel calmer and more trusting means strengthening your smart vagus so that it can tell your sympathetic and parasympathetic nervous systems when it's okay to calm down.

You can improve vagal tone by working on one, two, or three of these goals:

1. Starve some of the pathways to your sympathetic nervous system. An overactive sympathetic nervous system hogs all the stimulation, leaving the smart vagus with fewer opportunities to develop.
2. Strengthen the smart vagus directly.
3. If necessary, reduce stimulation to the parasympathetic nervous system. In rare cases, people equate social interaction with life-threatening danger, and the parasympathetic nervous system tells the body to shut down and play dead.

Ready for some ideas? You'll find plenty, below.

Ways to Starve Your Sympathetic Nervous System Stress Pathways

Many of us suffer from overdeveloped stress pathways. This can be the result of trauma, but it doesn't have to be. An overactive stress response is a byproduct of our culture. From our earliest days, we're taught to be independent above all else, and that the only safe place in the world is at the top of the heap, with the competition crushed at the bottom. This is the perfect environment for activating your stress system. By the time we're adults, most of us have spent two decades building up our sympathetic nervous system and ignoring smart vagus skills, like learning to soak up the calming effects of a trustworthy relationship. Adulthood brings a whole new bucket of stresses: paying the rent or mortgage, surviving life in the cubicle, raising children . . . not to mention worrying about terrorist bombings or anthrax in the mail. If you're living a typically hectic contemporary life with little time for relaxation and play, you probably feel chronically stressed. You're not sick, though, not any more than Juan was. Like him, you're having a normal response to a cold world.

And there was no doubt that Juan suffered from an overactive sympathetic nervous system. In fact, his sympathetic nervous system was stuck in the On position; he practically lived in fight-or-flight mode. That's one reason he was so prickly. Lots of people who frequently feel anxious are living with a noisy sympathetic nervous system.

If you feel so chronically tense that, like Juan, you are revved up and worn down, your most important job is to reduce how often your sympathetic nervous system kicks in. Remember the first rule of brain change: **Use it or lose it.** Use your sympathetic nervous system's stress pathways often enough and they bulk up. To reduce chronic jumpiness, you need to weaken those stress pathways by starving them of stimulation. Here's how to do it.

Reduce Exposure to Unsafe Relationships

Take a look at your relational safety groups. If there are any in the lowest safety range, examine these relationships more closely. Are you being physically or emotionally damaged by any of them? The first step to starving the sympathetic nervous system stress pathways is to end or reduce contact with people who are dangerous, who give your alarm system a very good reason to start ringing.

In Juan's case, this meant cutting back on time he spent with his father. I didn't think Juan needed to cut off the relationship completely, but together we decided that he could reduce the number and length of his visits. When Juan did see his father, he could bring Blanca along; he felt safer in her presence (that safe feeling was good for his smart vagus), and he wondered if maybe they could help each other by coming up with a plan to leave if their father turned nasty.

When a relationship is very stressful, it's not always easy to know what to do.

You should *always, always, always* leave a relationship that is physically or sexually abusive. If you are in a relationship that is emotionally disrespectful, the decision to leave can be weighed against the level of harm, the importance of the relationship to you, and whether you have other safe relationships to balance the emotional destruction. If the person who feels emotionally unsafe is a parent, the choice to leave can be extremely painful. You're biologically wired to connect with your parents. Cutting off a relationship with either one is like cutting off a leg: something you'd do to save your life, but only when there are no other options.

When staying is painful but leaving is too brutal, I suggest a couple of alternative approaches. Recruit a supportive mental health professional to help you with these. The first is to reduce your exposure to the emotionally unsafe person. Cut as far back as you can on the time you spend with him or her in person, on the phone, or online. Work with your therapist or counselor to help you identify how, when, and why you interact with this person. Those interactions are probably based mostly on the unsafe person's needs, but with some good help you may be able to change those terms. You can also start noticing when the unsafe person is getting worked up—and at that point you can end the exchange. As you get clearer about the ways that a person is being demeaning, and as you build other, safer relationships, you will be able to see the behavior and the damage it causes more clearly. This insight will help you make decisions that you can live with, including a decision to spend even less time with the person or, perhaps, to finally end the relationship.

While you're working to reduce your exposure to difficult relationships, you should also increase the amount of time you spend in your safest relationships. Every minute you spend with your most trusted friends helps heal the neural pathways that are being damaged by the low-safety relationship.

Consider Medication to Quiet the Stress Response

Aside from getting out of high-alarm situations, a smart move for calming an overactive sympathetic nervous system is to consider medication. Not everyone needs this step. But as Juan and I talked about how hard it was for him to sit still, he explained that he had once tried meditation. When he sat quietly for even a few minutes, his mind would spin, filled with traumatic images he could barely identify or remember. At this point, it was clear that he needed stronger help. He started fluoxetine, which is a serotonin reuptake inhibitor antidepressant, or SSRI. This class of drugs increases the availability of serotonin in the brain. You'll need to work with a doctor to get an antidepressant, obviously, and you should be aware that antidepressants come in different categories. Some, like bupropion (the brand name is Wellbutrin), can actually stimulate your sympathetic nervous system—which is counterproductive. I chose fluoxetine for Juan because not only does it treat symptoms of depression, it also buffers the stress response systems.

It can take between two weeks and two months for an antidepressant to start working, but when the effects did take hold in Juan's brain, they were very helpful. Juan felt a quieting in his body that he had never known—it felt like he finally had access to the ability to pause and reflect on his behavior. Juan reported that the effect was good but also so new that it was slightly unnerving. Now that he was a little less reactive, he could also sit still and even meditate—at first for just two five-minute periods each week, and then for fifteen-minute sessions four or five times weekly. When I saw him, he was visibly less jittery, and he looked less worn out. It was too soon to tell how long Juan would need to stay on antidepressants. Some people take them as a short-term strategy, sometimes for only six to twelve months; others need them for the long haul. No matter what, Juan had accomplished the first task: soothing his chronically overactive sympathetic nervous system.

Defuse Yourself Before You Blow Up

Do you tend to explode in anger? Many people with low vagal tone are on a short fuse. Juan frequently blew up at co-workers, girlfriends . . . anyone who happened to be in his sights when he felt stressed. But some people are like the husband of one of my clients: when he's frustrated, he loses his temper with himself. He doesn't lash out at his wife or anyone else, but his self-criticism is so vitriolic that it negatively affects everyone in the house.

Try monitoring your level of agitation on a scale of one to ten, with ten being a full-scale screaming, venting tantrum. The idea is to pull yourself out of a seriously irritating situation before it's too late. If you find yourself reaching a five, excuse yourself from the interaction. Leave the room if you can.

By keeping yourself from going over the edge, you decrease how many times your sympathetic nervous system goes into full-out war mode. Eventually, it will become less irritable and less likely to sound the alarm at relatively small problems. And, of course, the less you snap at people, the safer they will feel around *you*.

Relabel and Refocus

When your sympathetic nervous system is overactive, you feel more stress than other people. This leads to even more stress! Here's a way to step in and break the cycle. When you feel overwhelmed by stress, try the "relabel and refocus" approach. This method was created by Jeffrey Schwartz, a psychiatrist at UCLA who specializes in neuroplasticity, especially as it applies to obsessive-compulsive disorder (another problem with roots in neural pathways that have wired together and become strong from consistent use).[1]

First, for the "relabel" part, pause and take ten deep breaths. Stress causes us to take short, quick breaths, which reduce the oxygen levels in the brain. With less oxygen, brain cells can't work as well, and your brain becomes more irritable, which worsens the stressed feeling. So take those breaths—and then relabel your body's stress reaction. Instead of saying to yourself, *I can't take this!* or *My girlfriend is driving me crazy!* say, *This feeling is just my overactive sympathetic ner-*

vous system sending me a wrong message. This relabeling can feel stiff at first, or even ridiculous, but it helps you separate yourself from the experience of stress. This allows the cognitive part of your brain to come online and begin to modulate the agitation.

Then "refocus" your attention. Move it away from whatever is driving you nuts and think about something different, something that's pleasing. This is what Sally, the woman who lied to her boyfriend, did when she purposefully moved her thoughts away from how exciting it would be to tell a lie and on to how good she felt when she and her boyfriend were getting along on honest terms.

A particularly powerful kind of refocusing is what I call a PRM: a *positive relational moment.* A PRM is a time you remember feeling safe and happy in another person's presence. For me, a favorite PRM is the time I was walking with my then-thirteen-year-old twins toward Old Faithful at Yellowstone National Park. It's a gorgeous day and we're heading down the path, with me in the middle and each child holding one of my hands. Thirteen-year-old kids, willing to hold hands with their mother! When I bring this PRM into my mind, I always smile, and my smart vagus helps me feel less stressed. I also feel a fullness in my chest—it's like I'm brimming up with happiness—thanks to a little hit of relational dopamine. When I'm up against a stressful work deadline or stuck in Boston traffic, I think of this PRM. I know that instantly I'm activating healthy neural pathways and shrinking the ones that cause unnecessary stress.

(Of course, if you're stressed because you're in real danger, don't bother with relabeling and refocusing. Go ahead and let the stress response do its work—and escape, fight back, call 911, or do whatever you need to do.)

Relabel and refocus takes advantage of all three rules of brain change. First is the **Use it or lose it** rule. When you can lift your mind out of its stress, you *use* the stress response less; eventually you will begin to *lose* it. (Well, you'll lose its overactive, unnecessary aspects.) And there's the second rule: **Neurons that fire together, wire together.** When you are consistently overwhelmed by stress in particular situations, the neural pathways for stress link up with the neural pathways that pick up the sights, sounds, and other sensations of those situations. If you can keep these neurons from firing at the same times, they won't wire together as tightly. Finally, this exercise takes advantage of the third rule of brain change: **Repetition, repetition, dopamine.** You'll have to repeat the exercise to see results, but those results will happen faster if you add in the power of dopamine. By thinking of something positive, the way Sally did when she thought about genuinely intimate moments, you'll stimulate dopamine and help melt away the unwanted neural pathways. When you use a PRM, you're getting dopamine in an even bigger way, because a PRM generates dopamine from healthy relationships.

Try a Neurofeedback App

I've referred people with jittery sympathetic nervous systems to neurofeedback for years, but I didn't really understand the dramatic difference it can make in a person's life and relationships until a member of my own family decided to try it.

Ben was a highly competent man, admired by friends and colleagues for his keen intellect and easy way with people. However, his family and friends—and especially his partner, Aaron, knew him to be riddled with worry. Ben's sympathetic nervous system would fire, making him think that something dangerous was happening. He began to compile a mental list of dangerous things that could happen or that have happened—and the next time his body alarm went off, the items from the list popped into his head, and he immediately had ten things to worry about. Nighttime was a silent hell for Ben; he'd wake up with his heart pounding and his mind grabbing on to the nearest negative thought as an explanation. Unfortunately, every once in a while, something bad did happen, which was just the intermittent reinforcement his body needed to convince itself to remain on high alert all the time.

Aaron had mostly grown accustomed to the way Ben's anxiety could hijack their lives. When they traveled, he knew to expect an extra fifteen minutes before they left a hotel room, because Ben obsessively double- and triple-checked under the beds and in the drawers for forgotten items. Aaron barely registered the way Ben followed the weather forecast before a trip and constantly predicted that an impending storm would prevent their departure. Most days, Aaron could also screen out Ben's repeated attempts to feel safe and in control of his emotions. At least once a week, however, Ben's anxiety would surge unpredictably—and it seemed to suck the air out of the room. Aaron felt himself "catching" the feeling. As Ben panicked, Aaron could feel his own chest tighten and his breath become shallow. In those moments, the only way for him to manage was to leave for an hour or so to clear his thoughts and feelings. Ben understood Aaron's reaction cognitively, but each time Aaron walked away, Ben felt abandoned and judged. This chronic anxiety put them both in a no-win situation and undermined the relationship.

After his first neurofeedback treatment, Ben noticed a bounce in his step, and the rest of us, including Aaron, noticed that he was more communicative. After two weeks, his nighttime worrying had stopped, and even the daytime fears had greatly subsided. He radiated a brighter energy—and now Aaron "caught" this better mood instead of Ben's anxiety. The impact was so profound that he and Aaron decided to rent a neurofeedback unit so Ben could hook himself up throughout the week.

Neurofeedback takes advantage of the rules of brain change to rewire the brain.

Your central nervous system communicates by electrical current; individual brain cells send messages throughout your brain and body by electrochemical reactions. With a highly sensitive meter, the amount of electrical current sent through your brain cells can be measured and monitored. In an EEG, electrodes are placed on your scalp to produce a general picture of the electrical current running through your entire brain. The electrical signals emanating from your brain will vary, depending on where you are picking up the signals, and the frequency of current is divided into categories based on the wavelength and amplitude. It's the healthy integration of all the different kinds of brain waves that creates a sense of equilibrium or peace. For example, if you have too many alpha waves in the frontal part of your brain, you may find that attention is difficult. If you are having lots of anxiety, you may need to increase both alpha and alpha-theta waves.

Neurofeedback uses a reward system to help you pull your brain waves back into balance. What is so remarkable about this modality is that it bypasses cognition: you can't just think your way through a session. I was once hooked up to a neurofeedback machine at a conference in Texas many years before it became more popular. Electrodes were placed on my head in three locations, and at the other end they were hooked up to a computer system. On the computer screen was a game that looked like a simpler version of Pacman, one of my favorite old video games. When the electrical current in my brain gave off the desired brain waves, the Pacman unit began to munch up little dots. When my brain wandered off to another frequency, the munching slowed down. Miraculously, my brain knew that it should try to stay in the frequency that provided the dopamine-producing "reward" of the Pacman munching. After just a few moments, the munching was steady, the desired pathway was activated repeatedly, gaining strength and recruiting other neurons into its bulk. Neurofeedback is now more sophisticated, with dopamine rewards that appeal to a wider audience, such as watching a favorite DVD. When your brain waves are in the desired range, the video plays, and when they drift out of the desired range, the video fades out.

You can receive neurofeedback at a therapist or doctor's office, or, like Ben, you can rent a neurofeedback machine for your home. (If you rent a home device, you'll still need to work with a clinician to determine the appropriate settings, both at the beginning and as your brain changes over time.) But there's also an app for that: Xwave makes a headset plus app that you can use via your phone. The headset has only two settings: one that helps you grow the beta waves necessary for focused attention, and one for the alpha waves that you need to relax. The headset is a less sophisticated option than a full neurofeedback machine, but it can be useful if you want to focus on either of these two issues. Jennifer, the woman who felt a constant agitated buzz in her body, bought the Xwave app and headset to decrease her sympathetic activation. She often used it for fifteen minutes of relaxation at lunchtime—a smart scheduling decision in an office full of low-safety relationships.

More Ways to Treat Chronic Tension, Irritability,
and Jumpiness

Sometimes doing psychological work is hard. But teaching
your nervous system to calm down can be like a day at a
spa—wonderfully indulgent and relaxing. Even if these strategies drive you crazy at first (for example, you might find it
hard to be still), keep with them. You will come to love what
they do for you. Jennifer, for example, downloaded a relaxation CD. By following the soothing voice at night, she was
able to focus on each part of her body, first consciously tens-
ing and then releasing it. By the end of the CD, she was usually asleep.

Here are nine soothing suggestions for managing a
jumpy sympathetic nervous system:

1. Increase the time you spend with people who feel safe
   to you.
2. Work out. Moderate to intense cardiovascular exercise is best.
3. Use a relaxation CD. Some good choices include Dr.
   Alice D. Domar's *Breathe: Managing Stress* and Rod
   Stryker's *Relax into Greatness.*
4. Try the Emotional Freedom Technique. My clients
   report that EFT has a seemingly magical ability to

reduce the intensity of an overwhelming emotional state. EFT works by tapping gently on the endpoints of meridians (in Eastern medicine, meridians are your body's energy pathways) as you focus on the emotion that's been troubling you. For more information, visit the website www.emofree.com.

5. Meditate.
6. Play with a pet.
7. Take a hot bath.
8. Get a massage.
9. Ask a safe person for a cuddle or a hug.

Choose the ones that sound most appealing and see what happens. If you don't notice a difference after a few weeks, try a different set. Don't let these treatments go to the bottom of your daily to-do list just because they feel great. They're also vitally important to the health of your Calm pathway.

Strengthen Your Smart Vagus

Once you've calmed your stress pathways and you feel a little less reactive, you can start building up your smart vagus pathways. The benefit: you'll develop a better sense of when to trust people and enjoy them, and your brain will be able to send "relax" messages to the sympathetic and parasympathetic nervous systems.

Exchange Short Smiles

If you don't give your smart vagus regular exercise by exchanging caring expressions with people, it weakens. To help the smart vagus bulk up, trade short smiles with the people you like best. Not a huge fake grin, just a garden-variety smile that communicates a quick and friendly hello. Look the other person in the eye, and make an effort to notice the facial expression the other person delivers in return.

This exercise seemed like a perfect fit for Juan, who often avoided eye contact. When he did look at people directly, he often misinterpreted their expressions. A smile seemed like a smirk; a laugh might come across as sarcastic. In fact, when Juan and I went over what had happened when he blew up during the meeting, we pieced together the possibility that the junior colleague hadn't been trying to take Juan down a notch. He may have been more like a puppy, eager to share his ideas.

My instructions to Juan were simple: when you're interacting with someone, look at his or her face. Notice if the person is smiling or engaged in the conversation, and if they are, smile back and note what that feels like. This step meant that not only would Juan need to register the expression on the face of the other person, he would also begin to be mindful of the ways his brain and body immediately filtered facial expressions through his most prominent relational template—the one he had with his father. In that template, there was no kindness or respect. Juan could make a quick mental note that the person he was interacting with was not his father and that the smile was probably one of engagement, not rejection. This very basic process would activate his smart vagus and eventually improve its tone.

Juan began doing this with just Blanca and Bob, his safest relationships, but soon he moved on to his coworkers, too. Juan was surprised to find that exchanging a quick smile with colleagues gave him a momentary lift. Before long, he was able to hold longer conversations with people at work, and we moved our focus to helping him actively listen to their words. Engaging in facial communication and in active listening made him feel different—less alone and even a little calmer. This happened partly because he was enjoying the interaction, but it was also because he was, little by little, rewiring his autonomic nervous system.

In a workshop I did with a group of teenagers from the Bronx last year, we all took out our smartphones and looked at photos of smiling friends. I asked everyone to pay attention to what they were feeling in their bodies, and every single person reported feeling calmer, happier, or less stressed. It's amazing that such a quick relational intervention makes an immediately noticeable difference. So build a photo gallery on your desk or phone, with pictures of your safest people looking happy or goofy. Make a point of looking at them a few times each day to buff up your smart vagus and to feel better.

This is one of those exercises that can sound incredibly silly—*if* you have been told all your life that other people are judgmental, frightening, and competitive with you. Try it anyway. This is neuroscience, people; our brains are wired to work better when our faces engage and connect with the faces of others.

Listen Yourself into Safety

When a soothing sound wave enters your inner ear, the vibrations move the bones and muscles, and the smart vagus fires, helping you feel less stressed. So one way to grow the smart vagus is to listen to the voice of someone you love. You can also listen to music that reminds you of being with that person. (No breakup songs allowed!) The more you stimulate the smart vagus, the stronger it will get.

Another way to stimulate the smart vagus is to actively listen to another person. The next time you're feeling anxious in a social situation, use this technique:

First, scan your body and determine your stress level. If you pick up on a lot of stress, remind yourself not to talk mindlessly, space out, or walk away. Those are all stress reactions. Instead, try actively listening to a specific conversation.

In power-over cultures like ours, inserting your point of view into a conversation is seen as more valuable than listening to others, so it's normal to feel pressure to talk. But real dialogue means speaking *and* listening. It is essential to practice and value both skills equally. Take the pressure to speak off yourself, and head into the conversation focused on listening.

However, even when you no longer feel pressure to talk, listening can be hard work, especially when you're anxious. Your body could be screaming at you to *do something*, and listening means staying pretty still. It helps to give yourself tasks to focus on, so remind yourself to look at the speaker and mentally repeat her words (just in your head). If you catch yourself preparing what you'll say next while she's talking, gently move your mind from your own thoughts and place them back on the speaker. Ask questions, too, but just for clarification. Then run a quick repeat scan of your stress level. You should notice a difference; if not, go back to your active listening.

Ironically, actively listening makes you feel less stressed, and this means you'll have better access to the thinking part of your brain. When you do speak, you'll contribute more meaningfully to the conversation. None of us is particularly fluent when we're anxious.

Relational Mindfulness

Relational mindfulness is a two-person exercise developed by Janet Surrey and Natalie Eldridge, faculty members at the Jean Baker Miller Institute. It is a form of Insight Dialogue Meditation, and it is a powerful way to stimulate your smart vagus nerve by combining relationships with the known calming benefits of meditation.

Most meditation exercises involve sitting alone or in a

group, focusing on your breathing and attempting to escort random thoughts out of consciousness. Some types of meditation use mantras or chanting. The goal of these practices is to settle down your sympathetic nervous system by tapping into your parasympathetic nervous system. (Yes, some people have a freeze response caused by the parasympathetic nervous system. But for most of us, stimulating the parasympathetic nervous system in appropriate amounts and at appropriate times simply leads to a calm, centered feeling.) Studies have shown that regular meditation actually changes brain structure and creates more activity in the prefrontal cortex, an area that feeds back to the limbic system, causing you to feel less stressed.

Relational mindfulness uses the same techniques as meditation: breathing and ushering thoughts from the mind. But Jan and Natalie ask people to meditate by sitting across from each another, eyes open.

I bet this sounds overstimulating, and in some cases it can be. There's some evidence that when people hold eye contact for more than three seconds, they either fight or make love. Either of these activities will disturb your meditation! But glaring, unbroken eye contact is not the point. This is not a stare-me-down contest. A gentle, respectful gaze works much better, and you're always free to look away and take a break. Sometimes I have people ease into this exercise by practicing a few minutes of compassion meditation, which you can learn about on page 206.

Choose one of your safest friends to invite into a relational mindfulness practice. The first five or ten minutes can produce intense feeling; expect to temporarily Ping-Pong back and forth between activating your smart vagus (and feeling relaxed) and activating your sympathetic nervous system (and feeling like you want to jump up and run away). You may get a case of the giggles, too. But if you stay with it for just ten minutes, the stress of the interaction will give way to a safe sense of being intentionally held deeply and respectfully in a human relationship. The result can be a profound stimulation and reworking of the smart vagus, especially if you practice on a regular basis.

This exercise can be particularly moving and intense if you try it with a romantic partner—but do this only if the relationship is a safe one. Over time, a relational mindfulness practice can help couples bypass their usual squabbles. It also helps create even more safety inside the relationship, because the exercise trains the smart vagus nerves to fire at the sight of a partner's face. This leads to a calm, balanced feeling.

Starve the "Freeze" Response

People with a supersensitive parasympathetic nervous system feel so threatened by social interactions that they feel like they might die. I'm not exaggerating. Of course, they *know* they're not going to die, but their brains don't. Their brains remember an old equation: people = terror. It reacts by telling the body to shut down. This is different, really different, from the fight-or-flight response. It's a completely different branch of the nervous system that's activated. Instead of feeling a rush of adrenaline, you feel numb, quiet, and sleepy. You may not be able to speak if you feel this way. You may instinctively wander away and even feel like curling up into a ball. What you're experiencing is the human equivalent of playing dead, meant to persuade the threatening person to move away from you. You can't even talk to anyone to tell them how frightened you are, so people might react to your behavior by raising their voices or stomping around in bewilderment—which only increases your fear.

To recover from the effects of a parasympathetic nervous system response, you'll have to dig deep. Your body may order you to shut down, but you have to reach a compromise with your instincts. Go ahead and remove yourself from the situation that is scaring you, but try not to lie down or curl up. This is a time when you actually need to stimulate your sympathetic nervous system; studies show that mild to moderate stimulation of your fight-or-flight response can be energizing and focusing. But you need to stimulate it *gently*, just enough to feel alive and to warm you out of your frozen state. Physical movement is ideal—nothing very strenuous, just a walk, some flowing yoga postures, or even a slow jog.

A parasympathetic nervous system freeze response is a sign that you feel extremely threatened. No matter what the circumstances, if you experience a parasympathetic nervous system freeze response, you need more help and support than you're getting. Call on your safest friends and find a caring therapist who can help you gently address the source of your fears.

Take the Next Step

A feeling of calm is the cornerstone of a relationship. Without the experience of trusting each other, facing each other respectfully, looking at each other's facial expressions, finding the words to explain your relational experience, and having the patience and ability to actively listen to the other's point of view, the relationship can't feel safe. As you work on your Calm pathway, expect the positive effects to spill over into all your relationships—and into your other pathways for connection.

If you've practiced the exercises here and are noticing a change in how you feel around people, that's wonderful. Before you move on with the program, retake the C.A.R.E. relational assessment. Your scores may be different now, and you can adjust your next steps accordingly. Just don't stop! You've taken some relational hits in your life, but now you can feel even better by working on the next step. If you're following the program the way I've laid it out here, you'll move on to the Accepted pathway. But—of course—feel free to use whatever part of the program calls out to you. Always, the C.A.R.E. plan is all about *you*—and your relationships.

Chapter 6

A IS FOR ACCEPTED

Soothe the Dorsal Anterior Cingulate Cortex

*Here's how you feel when a relationship soothes the Accepted
   pathway:*
In this relationship, I feel calm.
I can count on this person to help me out in an emergency.
In this relationship, it's safe to acknowledge our differences.
When I am with this person, I feel a sense of belonging.
Despite our different roles, we treat each other as equals.
I feel valued in this relationship.
There is give and take in this relationship.

A few years ago, one of my fire alarms started going off at
random. I'd be in the kitchen or just walking down the
hall when the alarm would sound; each time, my body reacted

with a jolt of adrenaline and I'd rush through the house, look-ing for smoke. When I found nothing burning, I'd worry that an electrical fire was smoldering within a wall. Then one day I was so frustrated by the beeping alarm that I took the little box down from the ceiling and opened it up. Inside, I discov-ered a bug, cooked to a crisp. It had crawled into the alarm and caused a short circuit.

Having an overactive dACC is like having a bug crawl into your fire alarm. Remember the dACC? It's that small strip of brain tissue that activates when you're in pain. The Cyberball study at UCLA, the one where volunteers were gradually left out of an online game of catch, showed that the dACC fires when you're physically hurt but also when you're socially left out. As a species, we seem to be incredibly sensitive to being left out. Later studies using Cyberball showed that even when the volunteer subjects believed that the other players were part of a group they didn't respect, such as the Ku Klux Klan, or when they were told that the other "players" were actually a computer program, research subjects still smarted from the rejection. It's as if your ner-vous system understands that belonging to a group is crucial to your well-being; when you don't feel a sense of belonging, your nervous system wants you to feel uncomfortable, even wounded, so that you can recognize that you have a problem and do something about it.

But if your dACC has become highly sensitized, it sends distress signals at inappropriate times, just like my fire alarm did. With an overactive dACC, you're always worried about or running from social "fires," never feeling safe in a relationship. The process leaves you feeling alone and abandoned. These feelings of estrangement feed back into the dACC, causing it to be even more active in sensing social rejection.

It took a while before I understood that my fire alarm wasn't telling me that I had a fire; it was trying to tell me there was a bug in the circuit. It's the same for people with highly reactive dACCs. It can be hard to identify what's really causing your feeling of distress. Is it that people are excluding you? It could be. We live in a society based on social competition and on identifying the people who are "in" and people who are "out." Both children and adults get rejected, judged, and jostled out of groups all the time. It hurts to be excluded, even if we pretend that it doesn't. Just to make things harder for all of us, however, a feeling of social pain can also be caused by a bug in the system. It's easier to identify this bug if you know what to look for.

I traced the feeling of a "bug in the system" with my patient Kara, but it was a long time before either of us could figure out what was going on. She didn't talk about alarms or fear or pain (or bugs) at all. When Kara and I first met, she described feeling like a black hole was inside her. Sometimes the black hole churned like an active volcano; other times it felt like a dead, stagnant space. Always the black hole was with her, like a negative energy that drained her. Kara had spent much of her life in therapy, trying to extricate, reshape, and even befriend this deep, dark energy. Nothing had helped.

Kara understood from her years in therapy that this black hole had probably been formed in childhood, when she had experienced losses that were sudden and frequent. Her parents had been doctors who worked for a medical relief organization; they moved around so often that all friendships stayed fairly superficial. She could remember longing to be close with her parents, but for years the Vietnam War got in the way. Her parents were preoccupied by their relief work, the number of soldiers and civilians dying every month, and by their opposition to both the draft and the war itself. In Kara's mind, her early years were a swirl of tension, grief, and being on the move, although nobody really talked about these issues with her. Then, when Kara was in elementary school, her much older sister died in a car accident in a foreign country. Her parents pulled away from their remaining children, emotionally out of reach, where they stayed.

Kara grew into a woman whose life looked pretty darn good, at least from the outside. For starters, she was the vice president of a real estate investment firm. She had married and divorced amicably, raising a son and two daughters on her own. She talked with her children frequently and was proud of their growing maturity and independence. Despite her stressful upbringing, Kara had stayed in regular, though not close, contact with her two younger siblings; in fact, she often organized vacations with them for the express purpose of fostering connections. She had a vast network of friends and dated occasionally. Despite Kara's success and her connections, the black hole remained, and it ate away at her. She instinctively turned to her friends to give her relief from the bad feeling—and this worked, but only temporarily. Within an hour after she returned home from socializing, the black hole would reemerge.

"Relationships are like drinking salt water," she told me. When I looked puzzled, she explained that she could drink and drink, but her thirst was never quenched.

Kara's nerves were so frayed that we agreed to work on her Calm pathway to soothe her hypersensitive sympathetic nervous system. After a while, she felt brighter—but even a steady program of antidepressants, neurofeedback, and other exercises did not seem to change some deep, broken place inside her. The black hole was a useful metaphor for her pain, but I wondered what specifically in her neurological wiring kept this black hole perpetually intact.

Then something surprising happened. Kara was standing in the foyer of her center-entry Colonial, a house nestled in a neighborhood that had been home to centuries of American patriots, politicians, and business leaders. Waiters passed roast beef on toast points; from another room, she heard a pop and then a cheer as someone opened a bottle of Champagne. She was having a party for her colleagues and important clients. There, in her sparkling home, surrounded by history, celebrating with some of her favorite people, Kara understood for the first time that *she did not feel that she belonged here*. This feeling was familiar, but it puzzled her, because she knew that her own credentials were rock solid and that her friendships were real. Why would she feel this way? Moreover, she asked, *why would this feeling bother her so much?*

In an attempt to help her understand the particular pain she was feeling, I described the Cyberball research that tells us why it hurts to be left out. Naomi Eisenberger and Matthew Lieberman, who conducted the original Cyberball research, used the results of their experiments as the basis for SPOT, or *social pain overlap theory*. SPOT describes the "overlap" between the pain of being physically hurt and the pain of being left out. In our bodies, there is literally no distinction between the two. For people, being part of a group is essential, and being excluded is dangerous.

Kara's insight at the party grew into a transformative concept that finally gave the black hole a definition. The black hole was, in fact, a deep sense of never belonging. She'd never felt that she truly belonged to any group. In her childhood, Kara's family was disorganized at best and then, after the death of her sister, emotionally incoherent. Then she'd entered a mostly male profession, where she never felt that she belonged, and when she was married she never felt like part of her husband's extended family. She moved to the East Coast but never quite assimilated into its clubby culture. She had always protected her children from knowing about the black hole; she was unable to share her full experience with them. On it went, this feeling of exclusion.

The next surprise happened when we talked about whether this view was accurate. Did she always feel left out, or was there anywhere in her life now where she felt comforted and like she belonged? Her answer was quick and clear. Kara's two Burmese cats, Wellington and Sealy, were constant, warm, loving creatures who made her feel far better than people ever could. As she described her cats, she could feel the dark hole getting smaller and smaller.

There was another time when Kara felt like she belonged: whenever she was with her brother, Max. The two of them shared a familiar style of wit and good-natured teasing that was "home" to her. Her relationship with her sister, Charlene, was sometimes strained by their different life choices, but their time together also had this "home" feeling. Kara explained this realization of belonging with her brother and sister like this: "There's a feeling of 'Oh, I really do belong with these people.' There's an illusion that I don't belong with my brother or my family, but I do."

Kara suffered from a bug in her neurological alarm system. Her early childhood experiences of being left out had caused her dACC to become oversensitive. Even when she was included, her brain zapped her with painful messages of social exclusion. Understanding that her black hole had a name—it was the feeling of not belonging—and that it had a neurological cause gave her tremendous relief.

All her life, Kara had suffered from a social catch-22. She needed healthy connections to heal her sense of not belonging, but when she reached out to friends, her overactive dACC would give her another zap of pain. In effect, Kara's brain would say, "See? Here's *another* person who doesn't really accept or like you." *Zap!* Her attempts to shrink the black hole were actually feeding it. The fact that her friends actually did like and accept her didn't matter to Kara's dACC.

For Kara, the solution was to identify where she already felt accepted and to go there whenever the black hole made itself known. Instead of calling friends or making dinner plans when she felt bad, Kara would curl up on the couch with Wellington and Sealy. She'd pet them and they would flip over onto their backs so that she could rub their bellies. Or she called her brother. This was not necessarily an obvious set of solutions, because cats, however warm and wonderful, don't have the same potential for conversational intimacy that people have. And Kara was not as close with her brother as she was with some of her friends. But when it came to healing the black hole, none of that mattered. What mattered was that in these relationships, the feeling of belonging was unquestionable. It was simply there. The relationships calmed her Accepted pathway—for Kara, it was like putting an ice pack on her red-hot dACC.

How a "Bug" Gets into Your dACC Cortex

I've been talking about a "bug in the system" of people with overactive dACCs, but of course it's not a real bug. What's more, the so-called bug doesn't crawl into your brain at random. Something happens to create this effect of an alarm system that's yelling out the message *I'm being left out!*, even when people want to welcome you in.

For most of us, that something happens in childhood. In Kara's case, her nervous system was formed at a time when her parents were unable to give her warm emotional acceptance. Children desperately need to be accepted and loved by their parents. The sights, smells, and feelings of a parent's loving gaze and comforting hugs inhibit the firing of the child's dACC, and the more often this happens, the more that the second rule of brain change—**Neurons that fire together, wire together**—can shape the neural pathways to make this effect even stronger. But when Kara would look into her parents' faces, she didn't see a loving, accepting expression. Instead, she got a preoccupied or vacant look. This is not as obviously cruel as neglect or abuse, but let's be clear: it's still a form of rejection. Worse, it was rejection by the people she most depended on.

Young Kara didn't have the words for this painful experience, but over time she simply stopped expecting to feel anything other than left out. In effect, she learned that she was unworthy of loving relationships. As her therapy continued and the adult Kara thought further about the issue of belonging, she realized that whenever she started to feel a desire for more closeness to another person, she felt one of those zaps of pain. The pain carried a message: *What are you thinking, Kara?*

You don't get to feel close to other people! You know you don't deserve it. What was this zap? You guessed it: a pain message that began in her overactive dACC.

The Relational Paradox

When Kara "heard" her dACC telling her that she didn't deserve to be in relationships, she naturally pulled away from the other person. This meant that although Kara had plenty of friends, she wasn't really close to any of them. Kara's behavior with her friends fits into a pattern that relational-cultural therapists call the *relational paradox*. This happens when you're convinced that your friends won't tolerate who you really are, so you decide that the best way to be accepted is to leave a part of yourself out of those relationships. You think, *If they knew about my insecurities* [or past history, secret habits, or anything you believe would keep you from fitting in], *I'd lose the relationship.* Kara's thoughts ran along the line of, *If they knew that I don't deserve to be in relationships, they would leave me.* So, ironically, Kara tried to save her relationships by withholding her fears.

Of course, by hiding yourself you may preserve the friendship, but at a cost of feeling that you don't legitimately belong, that if your friends could see who you truly are, they would cut you loose. The more you participate in the relational paradox, the more pain you feel, and the more sensitive your dACC becomes—which makes you want to hide and protect yourself even more.

You can start to dissolve the relational paradox little by little. I suggest you start by simply becoming aware of the times you hide yourself or pull back from relationships because you think you're unworthy. This can take practice! Then you can send a soothing message to the place in your mind that feels vulnerable. You can do this by revisiting a positive relational moment, which I explain in detail on page 157. If you have a reactive dACC, it's useful to build a library of positive relational moments that involve a close and clearly accepting connection. Kara would say to herself, *Hmm, I hear my dACC telling me I'm unworthy.* Then she'd play a funny conversation with her brother over in her head.

Eventually, you'll be able to see your current relationships with less bias. You can even try sharing some of your hidden self with the people who feel safest to you.

Relational Problems: A Package Deal

Kara's relational assessment chart is interesting because it shows how one problem—in her case, an oversensitive Acceptance pathway—usually shows up in the company of other problems.

Kara's C.A.R.E. Relational Assessment Chart

Answer the questions on a 1-to-5 scale: 1=None or never 2=Rarely or minimal 3=Some of the time 4=More often than not; medium high 5=Usually; very high	#1 Max (brother)	#2 Suzanne (daughter)	#3 Charlene (sister)	#4 Nina (friend)	#5 Alex (coworker)	Total Statement Score	C.A.R.E. Code
1. I trust this person with my feelings.	3	2	3	3	2	**13**	Calm
2. This person trusts me with his feelings.	3	2	3	4	2	**14**	Calm
3. I feel safe being in conflict with this person.	3	2	3	3	2	**13**	Calm
4. This person treats me with respect.	4	3	2	4	3	**16**	Calm
5. In this relationship, I feel calm.	3	2	2	3	2	**12**	Calm Accepted
6. I can count on this person to help me out in an emergency.	4	3	2	3	3	**15**	Calm Accepted
7. In this relationship, it's safe to acknowledge our differences.	3	2	2	2	2	**11**	Calm Accepted
8. When I am with this person, I feel a sense of belonging.	3	2	3	3	2	**13**	Accepted
9. Despite our different roles, we treat each other as equals.	4	3	2	3	3	**15**	Accepted

Answer the questions on a 1-to-5 scale:	#1 Max (brother)	#2 Suzanne (daughter)	#3 Charlene (sister)	#4 Nina (friend)	#5 Alex (coworker)	Total Statement Score	C.A.R.E. Code
10. I feel valued in this relationship.	3	2	2	2	2	11	Accepted
11. There is give and take in this relationship.	3	2	2	3	2	12	Accepted
12. This person is able to sense how I feel.	3	2	3	3	2	13	Resonant
13. I am able to sense how this person feels.	3	3	4	4	3	17	Resonant
14. With this person I have more clarity about who I am.	3	2	2	3	2	12	Resonant
15. I feel that we "get" each other.	2	2	3	3	2	12	Resonant
16. I am able to see that my feelings impact this person.	2	2	3	3	2	12	Resonant
17. This relationship helps me be more productive in my life.	3	2	2	3	3	13	Energetic
18. I enjoy the time I spend with this person.	2	2	3	3	3	13	Energetic
19. Laughter is a part of this relationship.	4	3	3	4	2	16	Energetic
20. In this relationship, I feel more energetic.	3	3	2	3	3	14	Energetic
Safety Group Score	61	46	51	62	47		

Here's how Kara scores on the C.A.R.E. pathways:

Calm (add up scores for statements 1 through 7;
   maximum total score is 175): **94 (low)**

Accepted (add up scores for statements 5 through 11;
   maximum total score is 175): **89 (low)**

Resonant (statements 12 through 16; maximum total
   score is 125): **66 (low)**

Energetic (statements 17 through 20; maximum total
   score is 100): **56 (moderate)**

Kara's Accepted score is her lowest number relative to the scoring range for each category. But her other numbers don't look so great, either. She's only a few points higher for Calm—and that score reflects the improvement she saw after using antidepressants and trying neurofeedback. She had some trouble reading other people, and this went hand in hand with a low Resonant score. She wasn't able to perceive that others really liked her and wanted her to be part of their group. Her energy level was okay, but she tended to feel drained after social interactions, mostly because she felt rejected. It makes sense. Would you feel like dancing if your brain was telling you that you're unwanted?

These kinds of chart results—with low to moderate scores across the board—are typical for people whose neurological wiring is dysregulated. One problem leads to another problem that makes the first problem worse, and so on. It's almost impossible to know precisely where one issue begins and the other ends. If you head into a relationship with your guard up, certain that you won't be accepted, it's hard to feel calm or to project yourself in a such way that others can see the real you, and vice versa. Eventually, all your neurological pathways can suffer.

Fortunately, the reverse is also true. By improving one relational pathway, the others have a head start on getting better, too.

Safety Groups: A Warning for People with Low Acceptance Scores

I want to alert you to a danger for people with low Acceptance scores: if you don't feel like you belong anywhere, assessing your safety groups might be a painful exercise. If your groups don't include anyone in the safest category, you might be tempted to think: *Oh, look—here's proof that I really don't belong anywhere and there's nobody who really likes me.*

If you catch yourself thinking this way, stop!—and relabel this depressing idea as an inaccurate message from your overactive dACC. It may be true that you spend most of your time with people who are critical, judgmental, and unaccepting. You need to identify these relationships so that you can understand the damaging effects that they are having on your dACC and so you can start to repair the damage that's already been done to it.

It can also be true that past experiences with feeling outside and outcast may have shaped your dACC so that it's hard for you to feel like part of any group, even when people want to welcome you in.

Both issues—that the people you hang out with are judgmental *and* that your brain has trouble understanding that you are safe and welcome—can be true at the very same time. This is why sorting your relationships into safety groups is so illuminating. It can help you figure out which relationships deliver a lot of exclusion pain, and which relationships are more promising.

Like Kara, you might be surprised to find that the relationships you turn to in a time of crisis are the ones that actually make you feel the worst. This doesn't necessarily mean that these friends or family members are cruel and excluding (although they might be). In Kara's case, it simply meant that she had a fundamental, instinctive feeling of belonging with her cats and with her brother—and that these were the relationships that she could rely on to help her feel a healing sense of belonging.

Here's how Kara's safety groups shaped up, with a look at how she used the insight:

High relational safety group (75–100 points): None. This helped Kara further identify the cause of her "black hole" as a feeling of exclusion.

Moderate relational safety group (60–74 points): Her brother, Max, had the highest score and was the safest of all of Kara's human relationships. Her friend Nina also made it into the moderate category, but Kara's gut feeling was that she just didn't have quite the same sense of belonging with Nina. This was a relationship that she could improve when she felt ready to share more of herself.

Low relational safety group (less than 60 points): Kara's sister, Charlene; adult daughter, Suzanne; and her co-worker Alex scored in the lowest group. Kara tried not to dump her problems onto her daughter, who suffered from bipolar disorder and was often extremely reactive herself. Kara loved Suzanne, but the relationship struggled. Kara could instinctively feel a sense of belonging with her sister—but she realized she had to proceed carefully. Charlene wasn't entirely safe for Kara.

Alex was a tech wiz who ran the IT department at the bank. He often seemed emotionally cool. Kara wondered if he might even be on the autism spectrum. Kara concluded that her relationship with Alex did not hold much potential for acceptance and belonging, and furthermore she decided that this was okay with her. She didn't need to feel a sense of belonging with everyone. When she was with Alex, she knew how to identify the discomfort she felt, and she could immediately say to herself, "Oh, well. I don't feel accepted by him. Thank goodness I've got my kitties to go home to." Eventually, she decided to focus on accepting *Alex* as he was, instead of wishing he could be different. As you'll see, the judgments you make about other people can boomerang back in a way that heightens your own feelings of being judged. One way to calm your dACC is to let some of those judgments go.

Our Judgmental Culture Leads
to Social Pain

Kara's dACC had become overactive in response to her early childhood losses. But there are other ways that you can develop an overactive dACC. When a culture dictates that normal human development is measured by how separate people are from one another, everyone's relational templates are distorted, and everyone's dACC is reactive to some degree. To make matters worse for the dACC, we live in a hypercompetitive society that's always asking the questions: Who's prettier? Who's more popular? Who's a member of the "best" race, gender, religion, class, or sexual orientation? Who's more competent? Who has achieved the most? Who's got the best stuff? *Who's better?*

To a large extent, our social groups are created around the answers to these questions. This happens so unconsciously that most of the time we're hardly aware of it. Yet it has the effect of putting us all on constant high alert. A part of us is always scanning our surroundings, wondering where we rank against the people we see. Are we better? Are we worse? Imagine what it does to the dACC to know that we could be kicked out of our social group if we buy the wrong handbag or don't get the right kind of job, or if we tell our friends that we're gay or that we don't agree with their politics. In this atmosphere, the dACC is constantly stimulated— and then it becomes more sensitive in response. The result:

this primitive part of the brain is trapped in a vicious circle. The world looks dangerous; every encounter could potentially result in social peril. Then, in self-protection, the brain says, "Withhold yourself. Don't expose who you really are. Take the other person down first if that's what you have to do to stay safe." And then the world *does* become more hostile in response to you.

This is exactly what happened to my client Nancy, a fifty-something woman with stylishly tousled hair and a wardrobe of casual but expensive-looking clothes. Nancy wanted to be in therapy to talk about her relationships. She was worried that she was becoming more distant from her children and losing many of her friends. As we talked, she salted her conversation with judgments about the people she knew:

"Everyone can see that my friend's son isn't very smart. That's why he has to go to the state school."

"My daughter wants a promotion, but that's hard to imagine. She's so lazy!"

"Well, *someone* had to tell my aunt that she's annoying."

I have to admit: I wondered what Nancy would say about *me* when she left my office.

Nancy's harsh comments were the effects of a lifetime of living with a highly stimulated dACC. Nancy did not have a traumatic childhood like Kara's. But throughout her life, she and her family looked to "in" groups to satisfy a desire for belonging. Her mother in particular was highly attuned to how her children appeared to the outside world, especially to the people she wanted to impress. When she thought Nancy had gained too much weight or wasn't doing well enough in school, she could be bitingly critical. By college, Nancy was so accustomed to criticism that a relentless chorus of judgment sounded in her mind: she was too fat, too dumb, not sweet enough. Then Nancy fell in love with a slightly older guy who was studying for his Ph.D. He was ambitious and handsome and from an educated family. Here was a desirable man, valued by the kind of people her family had always admired. The fact that such a man could love her quieted the critical voices in her head.

Nancy married this man and started a family. They were happy at first, but under the pressures of new parenthood, Nancy's husband lashed out at her. She bought a new dress, and he told her she looked ugly in it. He fumed that she was a lazy mother who kept the children in diapers all day, when other wives were out working and contributing to house expenses. If Nancy tried to bring up a complaint about the way he acted, he turned it back onto her: "*I* don't ignore the children. *You're* the one who lets them watch TV while you pretend to get stuff done!" His attacks resonated with the words she had heard repeatedly as a child from her mother. Instead of making her angry, they confirmed her biggest fear: that she was unlovable. Her dACC pain pathways were being chronically stimulated and growing more and more reactive.

Plenty of people suffer damage to their dACC pain pathway as a couples relationship develops—whether the partnership takes on an abrasive tone or not. Falling in love is great for the dACC, as the two people pay extra-close, tender attention to each other. Although it's definitely not healthy for a partner to be as spiteful as Nancy's husband was, it *is* normal for the intense feelings of this initial phase to fade. If one of the partners has even a little bit of reactivity in the dACC, this normal pulling away may not seem just like a change in the relationship. It can feel as if the other person doesn't love him or her at all. The dACC becomes even more stimulated, and feelings of judgment and abandonment cloud the relational picture. It becomes harder to see the other person more clearly. All relationships take work, but the ones that are really close can be the most difficult, because there are so many opportunities for distortion to occur.

Nancy coped with her feelings of inadequacy by trying to fit in with the best social groups in town. She always put forth what she considered to be the best version of herself and her family and hid what she believed were faults. This was the relational paradox at work: in an effort to belong, Nancy was hiding parts of herself. Only the perfect parts could show. Unfortunately, her only other strategy for lifting herself up was to put others down. It was typical for her to "honestly" describe their flaws: her friends were told when they were being ignorant, unstylish, or just irritating. Everyone who Nancy knew was subject to this judgment—even her children, whom she constantly compared to one another.

When I would point out that a statement she'd made sounded overly judgmental, Nancy's face went blank, as if she could not imagine any other way to be. It was all she knew. Of course, her relationships suffered as friends, hurt by

her insults, showed her the door. Eventually, Nancy's relationships started to feel like land mines in a field to her, ready
to blow any minute. And when they did, she felt hurt and
judged and rejected . . . again. But she had trouble understanding the role of her own judgments in the explosions.
There was no template in her mind for nonjudgmental acceptance, no alternative to piercing criticism.

From a distance, it might be tempting to wonder what on
earth Nancy could be thinking. How could she believe that a
constant drumbeat of criticism would draw her closer to her
friends or her children? But that's what can happen when the
dACC soaks in an atmosphere of judgment. Judgment becomes the way it protects itself. Judgment becomes all that it
knows.

Exercises to Soothe Your
Acceptance Pathway

Social disconnection isn't just painful. It can have serious
health consequences. Science has long known that physical
pain stimulates our stress response systems, and now we
know that social pain is equal to physical pain. This means
that chronic social pain leads to chronic stress, too—and there
is an overwhelming amount of research documenting the negative effect of chronic stress on our minds and bodies. Stress
dampens the immune system and increases the risk of cardiovascular disease, depression, headaches, diabetes, anxiety,

asthma, and other conditions. People who live with chronic physical pain are at significant risk for health problems like these. So are people who live with chronic social pain.

Despite the link between social exclusion and devastating health problems, it's hard *not* to keep the vicious cycle going. Like Nancy, many of us are unable to see an alternative to constant judgment. Or, like Kara, we've turned the judgment onto ourselves, and the message that we're *not good enough* is so deeply written into our psyches that we don't even realize it's there.

The key to breaking the cycle is to become more aware of the cycle. It's so easy to pretend that social pain doesn't exist—that it doesn't hurt to be left out, that we're too grown up to feel bad when people are cold or rejecting. Both Kara and Nancy were perplexed by their suffering. They hardly had the words to describe what was hurting. That's why I'm devoting lots of space here to something I call SPOT removal, a series of steps designed to increase your awareness of social pain. I'm also sharing a few other activities that I use for increasing self-acceptance and acceptance of the people who are your friends.

SPOT Removal

SPOT removal is a set of exercises I developed in response to what researchers call SPOT—social pain overlap theory, meaning that social pain overlaps with physical pain in the same brain region. These exercises will help you identify how strongly your brain reacts to social exclusion. They'll also help you extricate yourself from the cycle of inclusion and exclusion that's constantly being played out in our stratified, power-based society.

First, think of a time when you were excluded from a group or uninvited to a social event:

- What were your feelings and thoughts about being excluded?
- What did you do in response to being left out?
- As you remember this time, what sensations do you notice in your body?
- What story did you tell yourself to explain why you were excluded?
- How did the experience affect your connections to people other than the ones who excluded you?

Then put yourself on the other side of the table. Think of a time when you, or a group you were a part of, knowingly excluded someone else. Ask yourself the same questions.

The goal of these first two steps is for you to become more aware of the impact of exclusion on your body and on your relationships. When you exclude others, or when you judge others, you are perpetuating a system of inclusion and exclusion—the same system that feels so threatening to your brain. This game of "in" and "out" is damaging to everyone who plays it. Even if you are currently "in," you feel, perhaps unconsciously, a sense of threat. On some deep level, you know that at any time *your* name could be called, and you could be the one who's "out."

I learned this lesson early in my career, when I was working in the psychiatric unit of a hospital where a clinician was being targeted by other staff members. The staff had some legitimate criticisms about the clinician's skill. That was fine. Being able to review someone's performance is critical to running an organization. But instead of giving her direct feedback, the staff turned on her. They made her the brunt of behind-the-scenes jokes and cut her out of the group. I'm ashamed to say that I participated. I was new and loved my status as one of the "included" doctors. A few short years later, though, I found myself on the "out" list. I was judged unfairly—just as I had unfairly judged my colleague earlier. Anyone participating in social inclusion and exclusion is in an emotionally precarious situation. Even now, when I think back to both those experiences as a young psychiatrist, my throat tightens and I want to hide. The experiences of excluding and being excluded are ones that can stay with you.

Repeating these two steps with a few different experiences of inclusion or exclusion will give you a better perspective on the revolving-door quality of this human dynamic. In, out, in, out. *Zap, zap, zap, zap.* Feel that? As you temporarily relive the stress of being left out, or the transient relief of being included when someone else is pushed aside, focus on all the feelings that arise. You may be surprised at their complexity.

Next, pick a time when you'll be out in the world for at least thirty minutes. Bring a notebook or your phone and make a small notation every time you make a judgment about someone else or judge yourself in comparison to someone else. When you're done, think about the messages that have been running through your head. Do you constantly think others are managing their lives better than you are? Or do you judge yourself as smarter and better than everyone else? Do you notice the weight of everyone around you, or their height, or the clothes they wear?

Judging immediately disconnects you from other people. In that moment, you can't see what does or could exist between you; you can only see where you rank in the power structure. If you've ever had a highly critical, micromanaging boss, the kind who thinks he's the only one with the "right" answers, you know what I mean. Every interaction leaves you feeling helpless, diminished, and angry! On the other extreme is the coworker who repeatedly apologizes for the work he's done, always sure that he's not good enough. He makes little eye contact in meetings; you can feel the shame he carries. The person who chronically judges others and the person who chronically judges himself base their interactions on old relational patterns and controlling images from the past. When you are in an interaction with someone like this, you may feel "unseen." Judgments are like a thick layer of fog settling between you and the other person, making it nearly impossible for you to see each other clearly. Some of these old relational images come from childhood experiences, but others are absorbed from the fabric of society's values. These are the "isms": racism, sexism, heterosexism, able-bodyism . . . in a stratified society, there is an infinite number of ways to judge others. Not only do we learn to judge individuals as a way for us to get ahead, but we also learn to judge entire groups of people and even whole cultures in order to justify an unequal division of power. By noticing how often you make mental criticisms of yourself and others, you'll become more conscious of the default program of judgment that runs in your head.

A way to decrease a chronically overactive dACC is to stop feeding it judgments. **So again, find thirty minutes when you will be out in the world with others.** When judgments pop into your mind, simply notice them—and then relabel them. Don't judge yourself for having judgments! Just say, "Oh, that's just my judging mind," and then actively lift your thoughts up out of their neural groove and move them to a new, more positive track. Try thinking something more generous about the person you were judging, even if that person is you. Or think about a happier moment, like your child's face during her birthday party or a relaxing afternoon you spent searching for stones on the beach.

When you take this step, you stop the revolving door of judgment in your mind. Active nonjudgments starve the neural pathways in your brain devoted to judging yourself and others.

This step is simple but not easy. The judging pathway isn't going to simply concede defeat and step out of the way to let the new thoughts take hold. The judging mind is an agile foe, and the judging pathways are robust from years of development. Expect some of the other neural pathways that the judging path has recruited to jump in and tell you things like, "But really, that person's hair is too long!" or "This SPOT removal thing is overly simplistic and a waste of time." It is essential to continue to notice, relabel, and refocus. Only then will you distance yourself from judgment enough to see that it isn't reality. Try this step for thirty minutes a day for two weeks, and you will begin to see the judging pathways diminish.

Challenge yourself to apply this technique in more complicated situations. Choose an environment that really pushes your hot buttons, like a political debate. There may be no place in American culture more judgmental than the field of politics (with the possible exception of fashion and beauty). Over the last couple of decades, opinions and judgments have become hair-triggered and hardened. This makes politics a great place to practice nonjudgmental acceptance. So regardless of your political beliefs, try watching a debate, or follow a political issue being argued through the media. When you feel a judgment coming on ("He's an ignorant idiot!" or "She's an elitist!"), see if you can notice it, name it—and then relabel it as the product of a judging mind.

Another challenging environment for most people is holiday dinner with the in-laws, whether or not politics comes up. So try to name and relabel your judgments next time you're sharing a turkey dinner with relatives who drive you crazy. To paraphrase Frank Sinatra: if you can practice active nonjudgment there, you can practice active nonjudgment anywhere.

The goal of this more challenging exercise is not to strip you of your belief systems. Having well-developed opinions is essential to a full life. The goal here is to create a healthier dACC by cutting back on how often you feed it the unhealthy food of demeaning judgments. And by starving the dACC in this particular way, you take advantage of the first rule of brain change: **Use it or lose it.** If your dACC isn't stimulated by judgments as often, it will lose some of its reactivity.

There's another way that toning down judgments can heal your brain. Judging is the domain of the emotional right brain, which is trying to protect you from something it perceives as a threat. This is a well-meaning activity on the part of your right brain, but it is an ineffective relational strategy. When you're judging, you're not listening. And if you're not listening, you're missing out on one of the best ways to stimulate your smart vagus pathway and turn down the volume of your stress-response system. But if you're not judging, you can listen more and feel calmer, and this, in turn, will make interacting with others much easier and judging others less necessary. As you listen, you may learn something new. Or maybe not; there is always the possibility that you will hear things that you don't agree with. Fine. Honest disagreements happen in even the best relationships. If you can have a passionate argument without pathologizing the other side as sick or malicious, your relationships will be more durable.

Sometimes people question the steps of SPOT removal, wondering whether giving up judgment means that they cannot give or receive feedback about interpersonal actions and behaviors. Actually, feedback is absolutely critical to growth-fostering relationships. How can you grow without feedback? It's instrumental in helping people see each other clearly and correcting behavior that undermines the relationship. But snap judgments and dismissive comments are very different from respectful conversation about what needs to be improved in a relationship. While both can be hard to handle, judgments are usually mean-spirited and designed to enhance your distance from the other person. Respectful conversation is in the service of the relationship. These conversations are in the category of growing pains; they are not fun to experience, but they are easier to bear because the pain isn't being held by just one person. It's being held within the relationship.

Judgments versus Feedback

What's the difference between making a snap judgment and offering helpful feedback? It's all about their intended effect on the relationship. Judgments set you and the other person further apart; feedback will, ideally, bring you closer. Here are some examples of both:

Judgments	Feedback
I can never get things right with you. You're never happy!	I try to consider your experience of things, but I am often confused by your reaction. Can we talk about how each of us can become more responsive in the relationship?
You're an undependable jerk for canceling our date last night.	Can I tell you something? We've been out on a few dates, and I like you a lot. But when you cancel on short notice, it feels as if you're sending me a message that your schedule is more important than mine.
You're lazy.	I've noticed that you tend to leave the room when it's time to put the kids to bed. I really wish you would stay and help me.
Your political opinions are crazy! You've been brainwashed by the media.	We have different political opinions. Why don't you tell me yours—and I'll promise not to interrupt or try to change your mind. Then I'll tell you about mine, if you promise to do the same for me.

What Are You Hiding?

Most people are hiding at least a few things—usually personal characteristics or beliefs or past experiences—from the people closest to them. Hiding who you are can make you feel safer, but only temporarily, because hiding produces follow-up thinking that goes, *If they knew the real me, they would reject me.* This is the relational paradox at work. In the hopes of being accepted, you don't share who you are—and then you feel as if you're always on the verge of being discovered and then rejected. You feel chronically unseen. What seems like a good, safe strategy for building relationships ends up activating your dACC pain pathways.

Ending this stimulation of your dACC requires some courage and at least one reasonably safe relationship. Begin by making a list of things you are hiding. Then choose your safest relationship and invite that person to perform an exercise in mutual sharing: you will both divulge one thing you've been hiding from others. The thing you are hiding is likely much more embarrassing or shameful to you than to the friend you are telling.

Here are some of the secrets, big and small, my patients have hidden from their partners, family, and closest friends:

- I lied and told my boss I got into a car accident because I didn't want to go to work.
- My family is from Germany.
- I took a year off from school after flunking out of college.
- I had an abortion when I was seventeen.
- I was sexually abused as a child.
- I hate camping.

- I give lots of speeches, but I throw up in the bathroom before each one because I am so anxious.
- Some days I'm so depressed and anxious that I can't get out of bed.
- Some days I really wish I didn't have kids.
- When I was a little boy, the older kids chased me all over the football field and I was scared to death.
- My wife earns more money than I do.

The relationship will probably be closer after you've been more honest with each other. Unpacking old secrets can significantly decrease the pain of life.

Root Chakra Work

In the Hindu and yogic traditions, the seven chakras are the body's energy centers, each located at a different point on the body and each governing a different psychological or emotional state. The root chakra, which sits at the base of your spine, right at your tailbone, helps you feel grounded and connected—to know that you belong in the world. You can try a very simple method of balancing this chakra by placing one palm over its area and another hand over your heart (the location of the heart chakra, which influences our sense of inner peace). You can do this while watching TV, meditating, or simply sitting and thinking. Over time, the bad feeling of exclusion will lift.

Compassion Meditation

Barbara Fredrickson, the director of the Positive Emotions and Psychophysiology Laboratory at the University of North Carolina at Chapel Hill, has spent her career researching love and acceptance. In her book *Love 2.0*, she describes what she calls "loving-kindness meditation" or "compassion meditation," a practice that her lab has shown to increase self-acceptance, decrease depression, and improve relationships.

To practice compassion meditation, find a quiet and comfortable spot. Breathe in and out, finding a slow, deep rhythm. Say these phrases to yourself:

> *May I live in safety.*
> *May I be happy.*
> *May I be healthy.*
> *May I live in ease.*

Then send the same wishes to a friend:

> *May he/she live in safety.*
> *May he/she be happy.*
> *May he/she be healthy.*
> *May he/she live in ease.*

Using the same script, send the wishes to a neutral person, and then to someone you dislike. Finally, send the wishes to the world:

May we live in safety.
May we be happy.
May we be healthy.
May we live in ease.

As you sit quietly, breathing deeply, you are decreasing your nervous system's level of arousal. You become calmer. When you send compassion to yourself and the world, you add a sense of warm-heartedness to that feeling of calm. You're teaching the brain to pair these two states of being—to use the second rule of brain change by wiring the two sets of neural pathways together. If your brain has been wired for snap judgments, this exercise will show it how to find pleasure in good wishes.

When you meditate on oneness and on compassion toward yourself and other people, you're enlarging—in a psychological and neurological sense—the knowledge that we're all one. It's remarkable to witness the change in people as they make a regular practice of compassion meditation. Over the weeks, its message begins to compete with the well-worn neurological pathways that insist *I don't belong.* A different pathway, one that has been weak for a long time, begins to remind you that you do belong, and that we are imprinted on one another. We can hurt and heal one another. And one of the best ways for us to grow is within our relationships.

Chapter 7

R IS FOR RESONANT

Strengthen Your Brain's Mirroring System

Signs that a relationship is Resonant:
This person is able to sense how I feel.
I am able to sense how this person feels.
With this person I have more clarity about who I am.
I feel that we "get" each other.
I am able to see that my feelings impact this person.

In a classic scene from the movie *Jaws*, chief of police Martin Brody sits at the dinner table, polishing off a bottle of wine. He rubs his face and his shoulders droop. There is no voice-over to tell me explicitly how Brody feels, but none is necessary. My brain has a mirroring system that takes in the information on the screen; it creates activity in my prefrontal cortex and somatosensory cortex that helps the neurons there internally copy his body movements and messages. The neural input passes through my insula, the little strip of brain tissue that helps connect context with emotions. This system of circuits from across the brain tells me Brody is exhausted and troubled. More than that, he is haunted by his decision to keep the beaches of Amity Island open after the first couple of shark attacks.

I'm not the only one who is mirroring Brody. While Brody is lost in thought, his young son sits at the table next to him, watching. Brody's son spontaneously imitates his father, rubbing his face as if he, too, were exhausted; he carefully raises his cup for a sip of juice the same way his father sips his wine. After a moment, Brody notices and plays along. He clasps his hands in front of him and then pops his fingers straight out, and his son follows along, pleased to have gotten his father's attention. The scene ends with a mutual, playful sneer and a loving kiss. Throughout the scene, Brody's son follows the actions of his pensive dad perfectly and mirrors his glum mood to a T. When they finally make eye contact, it's clear that Brody has been rescued from the brink of despair, drawn out of isolation into the loving connection with his son. That is the power of relationship and the beauty of an active mirroring system: one healthy connection can stave off the despair of shark-infested waters.

We are built to imitate people. Not because we are unoriginal copycats, but because we are blessed with a neurological system that automatically uses imitation as a crucial component of reading other people's behaviors, intentions, and feelings. The mirroring system can manifest itself in obvious ways, as when two people in conversation will start to copy each other's posture. You've seen this: one person crosses his legs and then the other crosses his. One leans forward, his chin in hand; the other copies the gesture almost instantly. I once had the strange experience of unintentionally copying George W. Bush. Just after he became president, his face was everywhere—on the cover of magazines, on the TV news, when I opened my Web browser. In most of the photographs, he was wearing that expression in which he appears to be in on a practical joke, like he's just put a whoopee cushion on his best friend's chair. For weeks, possibly even months after his inauguration, I would catch myself making the same face. And whenever my face transformed into a likeness of President Bush, his image would pop into my consciousness. The more I mimicked him, the more empathy I felt with him. The mirroring system is what allows us to resonate with other people without having to focus deliberately on the task.

I opened this book by claiming that boundaries are overrated. Resonance is the ultimate anti-boundary; it happens when one person's actions, intentions, and feelings are instantly, unconsciously replicated in a fainter way inside another person's brain. This replication is a good thing, because resonance is an important relational skill that lets us feel a deep-in-the-bones connection with others. Unfortunately, the mirroring pathway is the one that's most neglected when we're in a culture that emphasizes boundaries and separation.

Like the other C.A.R.E. pathways, the mirroring system is shaped by your relationships. It's well known that early, attuned relationships between mother and child lead to children who spend more time in social engagement, are able to better regulate their emotions, and are able to interpret and comment on their feelings and internal experiences.[1] The discovery that neuroplasticity exists throughout the life span suggests that pathways for connection, including the mirroring system, continue to shift and change in response to relationships. Healthy relationships nurture our neural capacity for resonance. Damaging relationships, especially ones with people who don't really understand you or see you for who you are, can weaken the neural circuits that are involved in the mirroring process. Those circuits may wither from disuse; they may not get the chance to build a rich neural network that allows for shared information; they may not receive the relational dopamine and other neurochemicals that solidify its pathways.

When that happens, it can be harder for the shared neural circuits that are involved in the mirroring process to imitate other people's feelings. As a result, you may find other people puzzling. You may think that everyone is blithely content when they are actually trying to send up flares of distress. Or you may be so sensitized to "dangerous" emotions that you *over*read people as being angrier or more distressed than they really are.

This oversensitization is what happened to Pauline. When I first met Pauline, she was waiting on a bench in the hallway outside my office, looking around nervously. Actually, she was looking for me. I was a few minutes late, and I immediately felt sorry that my tardiness had apparently increased her anxiety.

Most clients feel at least a little normal anxiety when they first see a psychiatrist. Truth be told, first meetings often make me a little nervous, too. I never know what I'm going to hear and learn. But Pauline's anxiety level was remarkable. When she saw I was ready for her, she turned her head down so that she was looking at the floor. I put out my hand and she extended hers limply, still without looking directly at me. As I said, her case is remarkable. I share her story here because it takes the garden-variety problems many of us have with resonance and magnifies them by a few factors, letting us see our own difficulties with greater accuracy.

As we went into my office and talked about the basics—where she lived, with whom, where she worked—Pauline relaxed a little. I tried not to look directly at her for very long, thinking that I didn't want to exacerbate her discomfort. When Pauline did look up, I made a point to smile and nod in my most outwardly interested way. Despite my best efforts to be welcoming, when Pauline spoke she often apologized about something she had said. "I'm not giving you the right answers, am I?" she asked. "I think you want more detail than I just gave. I'm sorry."

The interaction was confusing to me as we stuttered our way through the first thirty minutes. I'm an experienced psychiatrist who can usually get a lifetime's worth of information from a new client in sixty short minutes, but at this point in the session I felt like an unskilled dancer who kept stepping on her partner's toes. Pauline talked of feeling anxious much of the time, worried that others were angry or disappointed with her. Her fear with me and the way she described her disappointing and sometimes frightening interactions with other people made me wonder whether Pauline was unable to read friendliness on a face, or if people became frustrated by her inability to stay connected, make eye contact, and stop apologizing.

An answer arrived when we discussed her family history, and that answer loops back to the theme of early relationships that shape the brain. Pauline grew up with a father who'd gone to Vietnam when she was five and came home a brittle, angry man. I don't intend to point a blaming finger at Pauline's dad, because his behaviors as described by Pauline are in line with post-traumatic stress disorder—and this was a time when PTSD was barely understood, let alone treated. The mirroring system that helps you automatically connect with others does necessarily turn off in the heat of battle and produce an emotionally disconnected solider. In fact, I often wonder if one of the reasons so many soldiers develop PTSD is that, despite the adrenaline rush of combat, their mirroring circuitry reads the pain of everyone around them, friend and foe alike. That pain is stamped onto the soldier's nervous system. When the solider goes home, the pain comes along, too.

Life with Pauline's father was unpredictable. It was hard to know what would set him off—one night it was being served leftovers for dinner; another night it was the neighbor's dogs barking, or his discovery that the garbage cans were still out on the curb a few hours after trash pickup was over. When her father's anger began to build, Pauline's mother advised her to lie low, to take herself out of the tornado path of his rage. Just as meteorologists learn to read cloud patterns, air pressure, and wind speed for signs that a storm is brewing, Pauline learned to read her father's face for the earliest hint of anger. If his eyebrows drew together, or if his lips narrowed, Pauline turned and quietly fled to her room. I wondered if what had started out as a smart protective strategy—the ability to tune in to the physical minutiae of her father's expressions—had grown over the years into a hyperawareness of *everyone's* expressions, and the generalization that all of us were just a second or two away from exploding into anger at her.

I smiled at Pauline, and then asked her if she could see that I was smiling at her, and that I was happy that she was here, sharing her concerns with me. Pauline looked up and into my face. After about fifty minutes of talking about five feet away from me, I think this was the first time she felt comfortable enough to see me. She smiled back.

"I'm sorry," she said. (Apologizing again!) "I don't think I know how to do this right. The therapists I've seen before have always been so critical."

Certainly, I know a number of psychiatrists who would fit that bill. But I also suspected that Pauline had not been able to see her therapists and read any kindness on their faces. I mean "see" both in the metaphorical sense of understanding another person and in the literal sense of being able to look into another person's face. I paused two times before our session ended and playfully asked Pauline to look me in the eye for just a moment—which she did, followed by a deep red blush of shame. When I paused and asked her to look at me a third time, she giggled. This was a good sign and an important first step. This was not simply a woman with anxiety. This was a woman with a deep sense of relational fear programmed into her nervous system. Every uncomfortable interaction only made the fear stronger. Unfortunately for Pauline, every interaction was uncomfortable.

Let's take a look at Pauline's C.A.R.E. scores:

Calm (add up scores for statements 1 through 7; maximum total score is 175): **82 (low)**

Accepted (add up scores for statements 5 through 11; maximum total score is 175): **94 (low)**

Resonant (statements 12 through 16; maximum total score is 125): **71 (moderate)**

Energetic (statements 17 through 20; maximum total score is 100): **54 (low)**

Two things immediately struck me about Pauline's relational assessment. First, only one of her relationships felt even moderately safe. This was her relationship with her outspoken and ambitious sister, Maureen. Pauline wasn't 100 percent comfortable in Maureen's company, but she did sense

Pauline's C.A.R.E. Relational Assessment Chart

Answer the questions on a 1-to-5 scale: 1=None or never 2=Rarely or minimal 3=Some of the time 4=More often than not; medium high 5=Usually; very high	#1 brother	#2 Maureen (sister)	#3 Dr. French (boss)	#4 Leslie (secretary)	#5 Sandy (research assistant)	Total Statement Score	C.A.R.E. Code
1. I trust this person with my feelings.	2	3	1	2	2	10	Calm
2. This person trusts me with his feelings.	3	4	1	3	3	14	Calm
3. I feel safe being in conflict with this person.	3	3	2	2	3	13	Calm
4. This person treats me with respect.	1	2	1	2	2	8	Calm
5. In this relationship, I feel calm.	2	3	2	3	2	12	Calm Accepted
6. I can count on this person to help me out in an emergency.	2	3	2	3	3	13	Calm Accepted
7. In this relationship, it's safe to acknowledge our differences.	2	3	2	2	3	12	Calm Accepted
8. When I am with this person, I feel a sense of belonging.	4	4	2	3	3	16	Accepted
9. Despite our different roles, we treat each other as equals.	2	3	2	3	3	13	Accepted

Answer the questions on a 1-to-5 scale:	#1 brother	#2 Maureen (sister)	#3 Dr. French (boss)	#4 Leslie (secretary)	#5 Sandy (research assistant)	Total Statement Score	C.A.R.E. Code
10. I feel valued in this relationship.	3	4	2	3	3	15	Accepted
11. There is give and take in this relationship.	2	3	2	3	3	13	Accepted
12. This person is able to sense how I feel.	2	3	2	3	3	13	Resonant
13. I am able to sense how this person feels.	5	4	4	3	4	20	Resonant
14. With this person I have more clarity about who I am.	3	3	2	2	3	13	Resonant
15. I feel that we "get" each other.	2	3	2	3	3	13	Resonant
16. I am able to see that my feelings impact this person.	2	3	2	2	3	12	Resonant
17. This relationship helps me be more productive in my life.	3	3	3	3	3	15	Energetic
18. I enjoy the time I spend with this person.	3	3	2	2	3	13	Energetic
19. Laughter is a part of this relationship.	3	3	2	3	3	14	Energetic
20. In this relationship, I feel more energetic.	2	3	2	2	3	12	Energetic
Safety Group Score	51	63	40	52	58		

that her sister felt protective of her, and she mostly liked that feeling.

Not surprisingly, Pauline had been drawn to a quiet life, one without a partner or even any close, intimate friendships. She felt so uneasy in any interpersonal interaction that sustained relationships simply stressed her out. Pauline had chosen a career in science that suited her desire for quiet, focused attention, and for years, she'd worked as a research assistant in a lab. She loved plating bacteria on an agar plate and returning the next day to see what had blossomed. There was no reading between the lines; either the bacteria grew or they didn't. She found this work refreshingly clear, and she was devoted to it—she was usually the person who volunteered to stay at the lab after hours to complete a timed experiment or to finish cleaning up from a long day of work. So it was in the lab where most of her relational time was spent.

Her steadiest work relationship was with Sandy, another research assistant who seemed appreciative of Pauline's work ethic. Pauline also had regular contact with an older secretary, Leslie, who worked in the lab across the hall, but Pauline found her penchant for doling out grandmotherly advice "too much." It felt like criticism. There was also her boss, Dr. French. Dr. French was pleasant enough, but Pauline had felt that someone with power must be dealt with cautiously. She paid very close attention to Dr. French and could anticipate things that she wanted or needed. Occasionally, Pauline would curiously watch how Dr. French and Sandy interacted.

They were casual together; they even talked about their weekends.

The only other person Pauline spent time with was her brother, who could be a difficult guy. He was opinionated and bossy, and though Pauline felt loyal to her family, she also hated the feeling that he was always annoyed at something she'd done—even when she knew she'd done nothing.

The second thing I noticed about Pauline's relational assessment was that all her C.A.R.E. pathways were on the low side. In fact, her Resonant score was actually higher than her others. This was a measure of just how anxious, left out, and drained she felt. But it also reflected a few other things. First, Pauline's ability to read people wasn't completely off; it was mixed. She could study someone like her boss and learn how to please her. But she also saw anger even when anger wasn't there. In fact, her highest Resonant scores came from statements about being able to read other people. Pauline wasn't aware that she was *mis*reading them.

In order to unwind the relational knot Pauline was in, she needed to follow all the steps of the C.A.R.E. program in order. When the Calm and Accepted pathways are weak, people naturally become so preoccupied with their own internal fear systems, and by the relational alarm bells that are constantly sounding, that they are too distracted to see others accurately. After she felt calmer and more trusting (I thought compassion meditation would be particularly good for her— see page 206), we'd tackle the Resonant pathway. With luck, these steps would improve at least a few of her relationships and spark some good relational energy.

Not everyone with a weak Resonant pathway is convinced that land mines are buried inside every person she meets. Take my friend Dan, who's got a short fuse. When someone is distant or distracted, he believes that they are intentionally trying to hurt him, so he jumps all over them. Or take Darcy, who imagined—with pleasure and pride—that her employees and family lived in awe of her. She had a rude shove out of that illusion when she was passed over for a promotion and her husband threatened to leave her, saying that she had no idea what he thought or felt.

Ways to Tune up Your Emotional Resonance

What about you? Do you find it hard to know what other people are thinking? Are you often convinced that other people at work hate your proposals, only to find out later that they've endorsed your ideas? Do you often feel blindsided by other people's anger, which seems to come at you out of nowhere? Or have you noticed a subtler pattern of relational drift, of the warmth draining out of relationships that were once cozy and close?

Remember, if you have difficulty reading other people, it's not because there is something inherently wrong with you. It's a result of how your brain has been shaped in relationship with others. For example, if you live with a person like Darcy—the woman who liked to think of her husband as an admiring underling—you will eventually suffer the effects. When other people refuse to see your anger or your sadness, it becomes harder for you to see those emotions in yourself. In the vicious circle that by now should be all too familiar, you will then struggle to read anger or sadness in others.

Although your brain is inevitably affected by relationships, you're not powerless. You can take your neural pathways and reshape them. The exercises below suggest that you begin by spending more time with people who are sensitive to your feelings, and that you reduce the proportion of time you spend with people who can't see who you are.

From there, learn to label your own emotional landscape and then practice by trying to read the emotions of fictional characters you see on TV or in the movies. Other "safe distance" suggestions include limiting your exposure to violent images, which can overwhelm and confuse your mirroring system, and using the rules of brain change to starve the pathways that devalue particular emotions. When you're ready, there are several one-on-one exercises you can try within the context of relationships that already feel comfortable.

Spend More Time in Resonant Relationships

A while ago, I introduced the idea of relative relational time—that we have a certain amount of time we spend in contact

with other people, and that it's useful to know which relationships occupy the highest percentage of that time.

Pauline's relational time was spent like this:

Person	Percentage of Relational Time
Brother	25
Maureen (sister)	20
Dr. French (boss)	20
Leslie (secretary)	20
Sandy (research assistant)	15

If Pauline could spend more time with her sister, who felt
fairly safe, and less time with her brother, who felt scary, she
would leverage the power of good relationships to help her
grow. We agreed that Sandy was another promising friendship, and that maybe she could try spending just a touch more
time with her. Pauline started simply, by agreeing to make
more eye contact when she and Sandy were talking. Locking
eyes and holding the contact was too much, but Pauline could
briefly look into Sandy's eyes and then look away again. She
also used her observational habits to notice the kind of coffee
Sandy liked and left a cup on her desk with a short, friendly
note. Even Pauline could see that Sandy was touched, not an-
gered, by this gesture.

If you are in a relationship with someone who can't or
won't see you, reduce the damage to your mirroring system
by rethinking how much time you spend with this person.
Darcy's husband, for example, wasn't sure he was strong
enough to stand up to his wife until he consciously reappor-

tioned his relational time. He started playing tennis with a friend a few nights a week, and he began taking their children for frequent weekend trips to his parents' house. This was not done in the spirit of running from his difficulties. Instead, it helped him spend time with people who "got" his emotions, quirks, and personality tics. Eventually, he could remember what anger feels and looks like—and he realized that he was angry enough to have a healthy confrontation with Darcy about their problems.

Sometimes there's another solution: you can take small steps to improve a relationship that lacks resonance. I once worked with a recently retired woman who had become depressed and numb. Why? This woman had been an office manager, the bright hub of a busy medical practice. Everyone looked to her—literally—for guidance. Her mirroring system received constant positive stimulation. When she retired, it was as if someone had pulled the plug on this part of her nervous system. Her husband, who'd retired a few months earlier, had happily begun several painting projects. He was so absorbed in his new work that he didn't even look up when she entered the room. At night, he was tired and remote. My client began to ask her husband to say hello to her in the morning, to insist on conversational niceties that he thought were no longer necessary after so many years. After an awkward period in which their "Hello, how are you doing?" phrases sounded artificial, some of the neural pathways for their older, more affectionate habits reawakened. The person she spent most of her time with was now a person who could stimulate her mirroring system, not weaken it.

Identify the Physical Life of Emotions

Researchers have identified six basic human emotions that exist across all cultures:

Happiness
Sadness
Anger
Fear
Disgust
Surprise

These emotions don't just live in our heads. They have a life in our bodies, too, and even when an emotion is too distasteful to think about consciously, the body expresses it. Anger often lives as a pounding heart and rising blood pressure; fear can surface as chilly hands and feet. People who attend to these body signals and learn to interpret their meaning are better able to read emotions in themselves and in others.

You can cultivate your awareness of emotions in your body. It's best to do this in a safe and quiet place. Choose the emotion that you're most comfortable with, and then, with your eyes gently closed, let your mind drift to a time you experienced this feeling.

When I practice this exercise, I can easily generate a list of happy images involving my children. My son and daughter seem to live deep within my bones! One image that particularly captures a sense of happiness for me occurred when I coached my daughter's softball team. We made it to the championship, and my daughter pitched half the game. She struck out the last girl and the game was won. In the midst of a wild celebration with her teammates, we made eye contact. It was sheer pleasure. When I focus on this image with my eyes closed, I first notice that my chest feels full and that there is a direct connection between the full feeling in my chest and a smile that has formed on my face. I can't help myself: the feeling of joy travels throughout my body. My hands tingle a bit and I can feel my whole body energized by the memory.

Try on a couple of memories that call up the emotion you're thinking of. See if the feeling is experienced in the same location and in the same way—and if not, notice the differences. This simple exercise is one you can practice over and over again. The more you do it, the more easily identifiable your feelings will be to you.

Once you've practiced with an easy emotion, try a different one, something that feels less comfortable. For many of us, that emotion is anger. For some, it's fear. A sign that you're uncomfortable with an emotion is that you often read it in others. If people often seem angry with you or afraid of you, or if they seem so happy it strikes you as ridiculous . . . bingo. You have a valuable clue.

Jennifer, the young woman whose family gave her the

silent treatment, had learned over the years to squish her anger far, far, out of reach. So I asked her to let her mind drift to a time when she could remember feeling mad, really mad. And it was a time she was angry on behalf of someone else— when she first heard about the sexual abuse of young boys at Penn State. She was driving in her car, listening to a sports radio channel, when the news broke in. "The anger exploded in my body like a volcano," she said. "There was a bandlike feeling around the top of my head. My throat was so full that I wanted to scream."

When you try this exercise, you might notice that sometimes feelings are more complex and overlapping. When Jennifer lingered on the anger she felt, she noticed a deep heaviness low in her chest, close to her abdomen. It was a profound sense of sadness for the children. Jennifer didn't enjoy reliving this moment. But it was helpful for her to locate the feeling in her body and to know how to describe it. That way, she'll be less likely to be angry, or angry/sad, without even realizing it.

As you work on this particular kind of emotional intelligence, be patient with yourself. It took Rufus, who was addicted to Internet porn, about six months before he could identify the basic emotions in his body—and to notice that when something made him angry or hurt, he immediately zoned out so that he was no longer connected to anyone around him. As he got pretty good at noticing feelings in himself, I invited him to notice what I might be feeling. This was difficult for Rufus: first he had to actually look at me and then he had to notice my body language and facial expressions. We passed a milestone one week when I came to work slightly distracted by something happening at my daughter's school. Without being prompted, Rufus asked if I was angry with him. Instead of jumping to that therapy kickback, "Why do you think I'm angry with you?" I paused and said that I was more distant but that I was definitely not mad at him—just a little concerned about something at home. I appreciated that he pointed this out. It allowed me to refocus on the work he and I were doing together. In fact, we had a great session and I was so absorbed that I was able to put my troubles on the back burner.

Name the Emotional Spectrum

There are six basic emotions, but each of those six has almost infinite grades of intensity. Here are just a few of the words available to describe those grades, ranging from mildest to strongest:

Happiness
> Contentment, gladness, happiness, serenity, joy, elation, bliss, euphoria

Sadness
> Disappointment, hurt, melancholy, sadness, gloom, despair

Anger
  Annoyance, irritation, frustration, anger, rage,
  fury

Fear
  Worry, nervousness, anxiety, helplessness, fear,
  alarm, panic, terror

Disgust
  Contempt, disgust, revulsion, loathing

Surprise
  Surprise, shock, amazement, astonishment

People who live in an environment that dismisses the importance of emotions may have an intellectual grasp of each of these words, but it is hard for them to distinguish among these complex states in their own minds and bodies. Annoyance, irritation, frustration, anger, rage, and fury may all blur into one unnamable emotion. Overwhelmed, the person may express the feeling in an impulsive, out-of-control way—or stifle it.

Trying to interact with others when you don't have the full repertoire of feelings at your fingertips is like trying to run a retail store with nothing but one-hundred-dollar bills. With no variability in the denominations, everything you sell must cost the same regardless of its actual value. A pair of boots and a candy bar would both cost one hundred dollars. The boots may actually be worth that amount, but spending one hundred dollars on a candy bar is never a good idea! (And you're talking to a candy lover here.) If you have a narrow range of feelings, you may express an intense fury in an interaction when irritation would be more relationally useful. Juan, the computer programmer who raged at his coworkers when they commented on his ideas, comes to mind.

To sharpen your emotional vocabulary, try this exercise, which you can do in private. Identify one of your safest relationships, and then choose one of the six basic emotions and sit quietly while you imagine feeling the mildest version of that emotion toward the other person. Move up the scale of intensity. As you do, notice where you feel the variations of emotion in your body and how those physical feelings change. If you can't notice a difference yet, that's fine. As you pay more attention to where feelings arise in your body, and start to think about the words you use to label them, this important relational skill will come more naturally.

Next, recall what happened when you felt each of the emotional shades. Could you express them accurately? If you did, what happened next? In healthy relationships, the expression of emotions usually deepens the relationship—even if the emotion is anger with the other person. Jean Baker Miller said that one of the defining aspects of a growth-fostering relationship is that it produces a clearer sense of yourself, of others, and of the relationship. When your emotions are respected within the relationship, your capacity to form and express your experience grows stronger. So does your ability to hear the other person's experience.

You might try the same exercise and imagine feeling emotional shades within a riskier relationship. What are the differences? For bonus points, track a character's emotions in all their grades of intensity as you watch a movie or show.

As you repeat this exercise with other emotions, you connect your cognitive understanding of a feeling with a more differentiated sense of it in your body. Eventually, this will translate into clearer communication in your relationships.

Of course, the ultimate goal is to move this exercise into the real world. When you're with one of your safest friends, try saying something like, "You seem irritated/joyful/worried today. Does that sound right?" Naming the emotion and then checking in are essential. So many problems come from our failure to confirm that we're reading people accurately. Then we travel full-speed in the wrong direction, piling up misunderstanding after misunderstanding until the relationship crashes.

All relationships have a rhythm of connection and disconnection. It's impossible to resonate with another person all the time. The point is not to be perfect in your reading of the relationship but to be more aware of how you're reading them, and to check out what you're sensing. This is the **Use it or lose it** rule of brain change working its magic. The more you stimulate the mirroring pathways, the stronger they become, so they can help you safely span the enormous differences we all encounter in daily life.

Starve Neural Pathways That Separate
Feelings from Thoughts

Back in 1976, before anyone was thinking about relational pathways in the brain, Jean Baker Miller introduced the concept of *feeling-thoughts*—the integration of intellectual and emotional experience that's necessary for participating in healthy relationships. But in a culture that promotes separation as the goal of healthy human development, we're not taught to respect feelings. We learn that *thoughts* are the sign of a mature brain and that *feelings* are somewhat distasteful and immature. Unfortunately, splitting feelings from thoughts puts you at a relational disadvantage. Your experience of a relationship is largely based on how you feel about it. If you deny or misread those feelings, you can end up communicating in a way that is confusing.

For example, in my psychotherapy practice I often ask clients what they are feeling. Instead, they'll share with me what they are thinking: "I feel like I do not want to be with my husband anymore" or "I feel like I am done with therapy." The emotion that is paired with the thought is missing. One of the important tasks of therapy is to reunite emotions with thoughts so that the client can make statements that are more accurate. The statements become more understandable, too: "When I am with my husband I feel lonely and hurt; I do not want to be married to him anymore" or "When I am in therapy, I feel annoyed and angry at the focus on my drinking. I think I will stop therapy."

Improving your emotional literacy is a way to get better at communicating feeling-thoughts. The exercises I've already described can help you do that. You may also need to starve the neural pathways that are telling you to associate maturity with thinking and immaturity with emotions. Watch for these messages in your day-to-day life:

- Do you live in a family that says feelings are for children only (and preferably just girls)?
- If you talk about the way something makes you feel, are you teased or ignored?
- Are you in a relationship with a partner who criticizes you when you mention feelings, rather than just "focusing on the facts"?

When you are expressing strong feelings with someone who has difficulty forming feeling-thoughts, he or she may experience an uncomfortable mirroring of your emotions. The other person may even be flooded with emotions that feel unmanageable—and that's why the person may become rigidly fixed on keeping emotions out of your conversation.

Your resource against these messages of "thought superiority" is our old method of brain change, relabel and refocus (page 156). When you're in a family interaction and are criticized for mentioning your emotions, relabel the criticism as "simply a family belief." Refocus on a time when you brought feelings into a relationship and enjoyed the connection that followed. Or rely on one of your positive relational moments (page 157); I often refocus on my PRMs of rich conversations I've had with my children and when I do, I can almost feel the old pathways melting away.

Practice In-Person Contact

Are you in a relationship that's based mostly on technological interfaces, not in-person interactions? Person-to-person contact is essential for exercising mirror neurons. Taking in the sensory input from another person's expressions and actions will directly stimulate the mirroring system. The more interpersonal context you have, the stronger the neural firing along the mirroring system. If we're Skyping, you can see my face, and maybe you can see my upper arm moving. But you won't be able to see that I'm reaching for a cup of coffee on my desk. When we're not interacting in person, your mirroring system doesn't get as much information and won't fire as well.

Please don't give up on texting, Skyping, FaceTime, and the like—technology has become a basic tool for communication and keeping up friendships. But if you don't practice in-person interactions, communicating via technology will actually become harder. Why? Because when you have well-connected, robust C.A.R.E. pathways, you are able to read a few words from another person or see just his or her face and be reminded, both mentally and physically, of everything you know about that person. You have a context for under-standing the limited information you're getting via the tech interface. But if you don't have the body experience of the rela-tionship, you have to rely on *other* body relationships to help you decode the words or sights. It's like getting a message from your best friend but reading it as if it came from your mother—which leaves lots of room for misunderstanding.

Reduce Your Exposure to Violent Imagery

Violent imagery is ubiquitous—in games, the news, movies, and television shows. What's damaging about this imagery is that it rarely shows the effects of the violence on the victims. When we have hurt someone, our brains and bodies need to see the impact of that pain on the other person. Seeing the impact of violence and aggression on the victims directly stimulates your mirror neurons, leading to empathy for the person who has been hurt. In fact, standing in another per-son's shoes, or imagining what their experience is like, is an essential part of violence prevention and is the core part of most programs that treat male perpetrators of violence. But disembodied violence is unrealistic and does a disservice to us all. Marco Iacoboni says that

> taken together, the findings from laboratory studies, cor-relation studies, and longitudinal studies all support the

hypothesis that media violence induces imitative violence. In fact, the statistical "effect size"—a measure of the strength of the relationship between two variables—for media violence and aggression far exceeds the effect size of passive smoking and lung cancer, or calcium intake and bone mass or asbestos exposure and cancer.[2]

Being exposed to large-scale violence can alter the adult nervous system, but for children the effect is even worse. They are in the critical period of learning and neural shaping, and they absorb excessive violence without adult filters. The combination of the two factors means that violence becomes built into their mental constructs of relationships.

For these reasons, limit your exposure to violent images. Even I admit that some of the most violent films and movies are also some of the most entertaining—but for the sake of your mental and relational health, watch some comedies instead. If you're a gamer who is drawn to simulations of war or crime, try some games that are a little more playful or that emphasize collaborative activity. If you find it challenging to make this switch, remember that each episode of violence that you see is mirrored in your body and brain as if *you* are being violent or being victimized. If you reduce or eliminate that exposure, you'll feel better.

Know Your Relational Templates

Have you ever begun a romantic relationship with someone you thought was completely different from your parents—and felt relieved that, *this time*, you wouldn't spend your time together replaying the most frustrating parts of your childhood? Things go blissfully for a week, a month, maybe even a year . . . until one day, you wake up and *poof!*—your perfect partner is telling you how to dress and wear your hair. Last week she taught you the correct way to load the dishwasher, and finally, this morning, as you were hurrying to work, she made a suggestion about how to roll the toothpaste tube. You lost it. You had a full-blown, eight-year-old tantrum, the kind you used to have whenever your controlling mother bossed you around. In that moment, standing at the bathroom sink, it finally happened: your sweet partner, chosen for her laidback demeanor, had become your critical parent.

There is nothing more disheartening than traveling on these old relational loops over and over. But playing those loops is what almost always happens—because of the way we all learn to read each other's behavior. If you want to stop repeating old relational patterns, and if you're ready for some advanced work in reading other people, you need to become familiar with what are called *relational templates*.

At the place where your mirror system passes through your insula, there is a lifetime's worth of relational images, which are also known in relational-cultural therapy as relational templates. These are the ideas about relationships that you've held for so long you don't even recognize them. Relational templates are the molds for your ideas about how relationships are supposed to work, what you're entitled to within a relationship, and what particular actions and expressions signify. When two people misinterpret each other, it's often because their relational templates are drastically different.

Because early relationships and experiences sculpt our brains, and because our nervous system is drawn to the familiar for safety (even when it isn't safe!), we all repeat relational templates constantly. These templates become the unconscious rules that dictate how you act in relationships and how you expect others to behave. If much of your experience as a child was positive, with rich, respectful, and responsive people around you, people who were able to listen to others and to speak their voice, who could negotiate and compromise, you are probably in pretty good shape relationally. The skills of healthy relating will be built into your brain and body: you are more likely to have a calm dorsal anterior cingulate cortex, a robust smart vagus nerve to help modulate stress, and plenty of dopamine from family and friends. And you are much more likely to have a well-oiled mirror neuron system, with the ability to see people clearly.

In a culture that values separation, however, it is common to form a relational template that undermines your ability to read others and to be in a healthy relationship. An example is the close friendship between my friends Rob and Mary. They met in college, and as they realized they shared similar interests, values, and life goals, they became inseparable. Everyone thought they should get married, but Rob and Mary agreed that having the other for a spouse would be like marrying a sibling. The friendship survived graduation, cross-country moves, first jobs, and Mary's marriage. Even though they were on opposite coasts, they talked weekly and texted or e-mailed daily. Until Mary had a child. Rob flew east for the christening, and it was during that visit that a long-standing impasse began.

In Rob's mind, Mary was over-the-top obsessed with her child. She couldn't talk about anything else. *You can put her down for just one minute!* Rob would think as Mary tried to carry on conversations with Rob about her baby—all the while tending to her baby. Rob knew that babies are adorable and that they require hard work, but wasn't this a little much? He was surprised to feel divorced from Mary's world. *Am I really jealous of a baby?* he wondered.

Mary picked up on Rob's distraction, but she assumed he was just consumed by a job he'd recently started. But over the months, Rob grew frustrated by how long it took Mary to respond to his messages and how often she had to end their phone calls because of some need of the baby's. And talk about the baby was a colossal bore to Rob. He grew more and more distant. Their communication faded. Both felt an enormous loss but had no idea what to do about it.

Neither realized that deep-seated relational templates were playing out in the way they related to each other. Mary had grown up as an only child and had loved every minute of it. Her mother had doted on her and still did. Every month or so, she'd send Mary a care package filled with all her favorite treats—this made Mary feel seven years old again, in the best way possible—and they enjoyed long, chatty conversations. Mary always expected that she'd be the same kind of mother to her own child. Who wouldn't make a baby the center of the family universe?

Rob also enjoyed attentive parents—until his brother was born with cerebral palsy. Rob's mother and brother nearly died during the birth, and although both survived, little Jonathan was disabled for life. The house was transformed into a medical ward filled with wheelchairs, special beds, oxygen, and medications to keep Jonathan alive. Everything about their lives needed to fit around his schedule. Rob knew that his parents still loved him, but they were so overwhelmed and tired from taking care of his brother that he couldn't help feeling left out.

In print, it's not hard to see how Rob's and Mary's experiences have formed two very different relational templates. But the nature of relational templates is that they're our only reference point for how relationships should work. They feel like an instinctive list of the things all people are just supposed to know about how we relate with others. So to Mary, it felt like "everyone knows" that a new baby is supposed to be the center of everyone's attention. To Rob, it seemed that "everyone knows" that when you stop paying close attention to your best friend, you're sending a clear message to that friend: bye-bye. Rob and Mary didn't realize that they were reading from two different scripts, so they were both confused and hurt.

The tension broke one evening when Mary reached out to Rob in tears. Despite their distance, he was the only person she wanted to talk to about how isolating and tiring it can be to take care of a child full time. Rob was so relieved that Mary still saw him as a confidant that he was able to step out of his anger and feel compassion. They had a long talk that night, each explaining what they'd been thinking and feeling. Rob was finally able to make sense of his anger as he described the pain of being pushed out of his mother's arms by a sick little brother. Mary realized that not everyone shared her mother/baby ideal. By identifying elements of their relational templates, they were able to see each other more clearly and compassionately. This is how a good relationship can shape your brain for the better. In this case, Rob's and Mary's mirror neuron systems were strengthened when they learned more about how to "read" each other.

Relational templates are a major reason we misread people. Rob's relational template told him that a mother can love only one person at a time. Pauline's template told her that everyone teeters on a knife's-edge of anger. Jennifer's template framed low expectations of how other people would act toward her; she hardly knew when she was being mistreated. If you build an awareness of these deeply grooved mental pathways, you can more easily find your way to clarity when things in the relationship become confusing or fuzzy. It's like knowing to put on your prescription glasses to correct your out-of-focus vision. And we *all* need these "glasses" to help us see others, because we've all internalized different relational templates.

Use Your C.A.R.E. Relational Assessment to Spot Patterns

One way to spot some of your relational templates is to review the results of your C.A.R.E. Relational Assessment Chart. Look for patterns that carry over from one relationship to another. For example, Jennifer noticed that she had only one relationship in which she felt clear about herself most of the time. Eventually she decided that when she entered into most relationships she would feel confused—not just about how to express her needs but what those needs actually were. She hadn't quite felt the pain of this confusion before, because her family life had taught her it was normal to not be seen, heard, or understood. One client, who'd just realized that she played the emotional caretaker for her group of friends, arched her eyebrows and said, "Well, *that* sounds familiar. And by familiar, I mean familial." Of course, relationships are not simply replays of past relational experiences; each has its own tempo and color. So each relationship you evaluate will look a little different from the others. Nevertheless, you'll probably spy some general patterns.

Let Friends Help You "See" Your Template

Minds can get caught in perpetual self-deceptive loops. ("It's not that I imagine that other people are angry," Pauline said to me, "it's just that nobody else but me can see how angry they are.") That's why you'll want to collect some information about your relational patterns that comes from outside yourself. Invite someone from your relational safety group to give you honest feedback about how he or she sees you in your relational world. (If you don't have anyone in that group yet, wait until you do. If you ask someone who doesn't see you clearly to perform this work, you could end up with a distorted view of yourself.) Most people are hesitant to offer criticism of their friends, so here's a list of questions to get the conversation started:

1. Am I always the one doing the caretaking?
2. When other people have strong opinions, do I defer to them?
3. Do I have a hard time listening to others?
4. Do I get angry when other people challenge me?
5. When there is a conflict, do I get hurt easily and withdraw?
6. Am I aggressive when I don't get my way?
7. Do I act differently with men than with women?
8. Am I controlling?

9. Am I often too scattered and distracted to engage with people?

10. Do I say things impulsively that hurt people's feelings?

Unlock Implicit Memories

Explicit memories are the visual, often narrative memories that you can picture in your mind. You can't start saving explicit memories until the hippocampus, the memory storage in your brain, forms sometime between the ages of three and six. When people ask you about your very first memory, they're really asking about your first *explicit* memory. Your implicit memory, on the other hand, is formed in your first couple years of life, before the hippocampus is up and running. Memories that are stored implicitly are thought to be related to the action of the amygdala, which is associated with emotions and stress; these memories come up not on visual tracks but as feelings and bodily sensations.

You may not be able to "remember," in the traditional sense, the times your mother pushed you away when you were scared, or the times in nursery school when other children made fun of your lisp, or even the moments of absolute peace and comfort when you nestled into your grandmother's soft lap. Implicit memories are not visual; they're more like subliminal background noise stored in the cells of your body, constantly feeding you information about what to expect in the world. They may emerge as feelings or bodily sensations, as when you find yourself flooded with a strong dislike for someone with no apparent cause, or when a stranger seems familiar to you. Because these implicit memories don't *feel* like memories, they become the "truths" we fail to question, our biases, and source of any rigidity we feel in relationships. They also feel like the essence of your nature, so changing them or even identifying them as having the potential for change can feel downright scary.

I can't give you a way to track your implicit memories to an external event in the world. But there's a way to track some of the "truths" that are triggered by powerful implicit memories, and to help you realize how relative these truths can be. Begin by recalling a time when you were in a seemingly unresolvable conflict with someone. What was the truth you carried into the conflict—the idea that you knew, deep down, was correct and just? When you can identify this truth, you can be pretty sure you're touching the tip of an implicit memory.

Now try to identify the truth you believe the other person brought into the conflict. And then—here's the hard part—imagine a bridging truth that would allow both realities to exist. For example, Rob and Mary were each eventually able to identify the truths they brought into their conflict about how people should treat each other. A bridging truth was that a mother's tight bond with her baby could be healthy, but that the time she devoted to creating that bond could cause the mother's friend to feel lonely. Another bridging truth was that Rob and Mary missed each other and wanted the relationship to continue.

The point of this exercise is not to change all your core beliefs but to bring you an awareness of how relative and experiential they are. Sane people can and will differ on some pretty critical life issues, and having the brain flexibility to imagine the outlines of another person's relational template is a key relational skill.

Starve Unwanted Relational Images

So far, I've described how to reduce the power of your relational template by becoming more aware of it. In this final step, you can use the rules of brain change to actually change some of the relational images within your template. Make a mental list of the relational ideas that form your individual template; note how you feel when a relationship bumps up against one of those ideas. Decide which memories, images, and ideas you want to hold on to and which ones you'd like to move further into the background. You can't delete your memories, but you can move them further into the background of your mind. They will still be part of your life, but they can be a part that has little relevance to your relationships today.

And it's back to the relabel and refocus technique to starve the unwanted relational images. When an unwanted implicit or explicit memory makes itself known, simply label it as an old relational image. By giving it a name, you're separating the image from absolute reality. Then call on the third rule of brain change: **Repetition, repetition, dopamine.** Every time you relabel the image, refocus your mind on an especially pleasant PRM. With time (that's the repetition part), the old relational images will fade. (For more about relabeling, refocusing, and PRMs, see page 156.)

Rob, who realized how close he'd come to drifting away from his friend Mary forever, tried this technique. His template had been formed by the feeling that people he loved would push him aside, that he'd get bumped out by someone who was needier and more important. His head told him that his little brother was sick and vulnerable—of course he needed most of his parents' attention—but the memories stored in his body told a different story. When he imagined that time period, he could feel his heart beating faster, his chest growing tight, and his whole body coursing with a feeling of irritability. He could also feel, just below the anxiety, a profound sadness. When he paid attention to this feeling, forgotten images emerged: before his brother was born, he'd been excited. He was going to be a big brother! He was going to show this little guy his favorite toys; they were going to share a bedroom; and when they were supposed to go to sleep they would stay awake and have fun together. The grief of that loss was profound.

This loss—which was a controlling relational image for Rob—had influenced his adult interactions. Whenever he would become interested in a woman, he would immediately say to himself, *Don't get your hopes up.* He didn't like to let himself look forward to anything; he tried not to put himself in a position where he could be disappointed. In fact, that's why his relationship with Mary worked so well. She was a friend, with no pressure for anything more to develop. He loved that. It felt safe. But this impulse toward safety above all else had almost ruined his friendship with Mary, and it had ended other relationships before they could get off the ground.

Slowly, Rob began to starve the neural pathway, the one that told him not to get his hopes up. When he met a new person at work or a woman he liked, warnings poured into his head—and Rob reminded himself, "These are the ghosts of old memories from when my brother was born; they do not apply today." Then he focused on how he and Mary had reconnected. As his relational images became more explicit to him, they released their grip; and as he devoted more neural space to the memory of diving deeper into his friendship with Mary, he grew more confident. There is nothing more powerful than realizing you've rewired your brain for more hope and happiness.

Chapter 8

E IS FOR ENERGETIC

Reconnect Your Dopamine Reward System to Healthy Relationships

*How do you know if a relationship stimulates your Energetic
   pathway? It feels like this:*
This relationship helps me be more productive in my life.
I enjoy the time I spend with this person.
Laughter is a part of this relationship.
In this relationship, I feel more energetic.

Take a look at this couple in trouble, and think about how
you'd describe their problems:

Melissa and Maggie sat on the couch in my office. Unlike many couples who come in for therapy, they were sitting
together, holding hands. But something was clearly wrong.

They looked more like tired colleagues at the end of a long shift than partners in love.

The complaints tumbled out. Melissa had started drinking. First one glass of wine every now and then; then a glass every night; and soon she was buying a couple of bottles of pinot at the grocery store on Saturdays, just to see her through the week. Maggie didn't drink. "I'm too busy," she said, a bit primly.

Melissa arched an eyebrow. "Not too busy to watch hours of TV at a time," she noted. "And it's *stupid* TV."

A backstory emerged. Melissa and Maggie began seeing each other in college, where each was hundreds of miles from her family. As the romance progressed, they started to spend most weekends together. Melissa was aware that Maggie was close to her family, but it wasn't until their senior year, when Melissa and Maggie moved in together, that it became clear Maggie called or texted them multiple times a day.

Which elective sounds better: Kinesiology or Intro to Theater?

Remind me what kind of tomato sauce Mom buys.

How did the twins' basketball practice go today?

Maggie rarely made a move without discussing it first with her family. Melissa found this odd, but not terribly troubling. The Melissa she knew was strong and capable, a woman who'd majored in electrical engineering and who had once told off the track coach for intimidating a freshman at practice.

The summer after graduation, Melissa and Maggie were

married. When Melissa found herself at the altar of a large, progressive church, she paused . . . and then she panicked. Glancing out at the church pews, she saw plenty of people but few familiar faces. Maggie's guests outnumbered hers by at least five to one.

"Hundreds of people," Melissa said to me, when the two of them came in for couples therapy a few years later. "And almost all were members of her family!"

"Well, who was I supposed to leave out?" Maggie asked. "You don't exclude family!" She turned to me for confirmation. "Right?"

It was an argument they'd had several times over. Melissa marked the ceremony as the point when her life became overrun by weddings, funerals, christenings, football games, and weekly Sunday dinners with her very large and very committed clan of in-laws. Melissa had agreed to move back to Maggie's hometown after they married, imagining that it would help them save money and give Maggie the emotional support she needed as Melissa started a career in finance with long hours. Within a couple months, though, Melissa realized she was leading her in-laws' life, not her own. The weekends that Maggie and Melissa used to enjoy together as a couple changed dramatically. Sundays in particular were all-day family events. After church—where everyone went together and sat in the same pews every week—they all gathered at the parents' house for lunch. They would eat a big meal that was served in the midafternoon, often with several courses. Then they sat around and talked and watched TV until night fell. Spending the day in a different manner was out of the question. In a broader sense, Melissa felt that Maggie's family was trying to suck them into their groupthink. At college, Melissa had enjoyed debating issues with Maggie, who'd held her own opinions. But now Maggie, her brothers and sisters, and her mother planned events together, painted their family rooms the same colors, consulted each other about what to eat for dinner, and were similarly critical of their spouses as a group—as if all the loves in their lives were an identical lump. The day that Melissa's sister-in-law came over to suggest some improvements to their front yard, Melissa broke.

"My God, your family can't let us alone! They expect us to be with them, all together, all of the time. It's like we've been absorbed by a giant amoeba."

Maggie lobbed back. "Oh, would you rather live the way your family does? They've only come to visit us once! And your mother didn't even give you a *hug* when she got off the plane."

"At least my family loves me enough to let me go and live my life!"

Since the landscaping incident, Melissa had refused to attend any of family gatherings. Melissa suspected that she'd become a scapegoat, with Maggie and her family bonding behind her back by talking about how different and strange Melissa was. It was about this time that the drinking had started.

Maggie treasured her family bond. When they were all together, she felt cozy and cherished. She could admit to some problems, though. Having expanded her beliefs, her likes, and dislikes during the four years away from home, she occasionally bristled at the way her mother tried to run her life. Often her mother would announce plans and simply assume that the "children" (all fully grown adults) would go along with them. Maggie had loved the independence she had in college, not to mention the togetherness she'd felt with Melissa. As they talked, a wave of missing Melissa swept over her.

"But there's the drinking . . ." Maggie said.

"There's your lack of interest in my *entire life*," Melissa said simply.

Maggie and Melissa are clearly at a crisis point, both in their marriage and in their lives as new adults.

What's gone wrong? What should Maggie and Melissa do?

This chapter is called "E Is for Energetic," so it's probably obvious that I'm thinking of Maggie and Melissa's problems in terms of their Energetic pathways, which transmits the feel-good, animating neurochemical, dopamine. But first let's look at their marriage in the same way that popular culture views couples' issues. Let's look at it through the lens of separation and individuation.

In this view, a few aspects of Maggie and Melissa's problem are clear. The first is that Maggie's family is pathologically unwilling to let her separate. If Maggie wants to do the essential work of growing up and forming a family of her own with Melissa, she will have to understand that her parents and siblings have been stunting her emotional growth with their demands for closeness. Their desire to have Maggie with them may look like love, but it's not: it's a desire to prevent her from growing into her own person, from developing boundaries between herself and them. If Maggie wants to survive as an individual, she will have to kick at her family, much the way a rebellious teenager would do, and push them away in order to recapture the independent self she forged in college. Only then will she be a mature person, ready to pull her weight in her marriage.

In this scenario, Maggie will have to forfeit the closeness and warmth she feels with her family. Would she be willing to do this? She might. If a trusted therapist tells Maggie that her family has deprived her of something that is essential for her growth, she might be so angry at her family that she'll *want* to push them away. If she feels she's been wronged, the loss of her family closeness won't sting as much as it otherwise might. One likely outcome is that Maggie will develop a kind of angry, amused tolerance of her needy family members. Instead of joking about Melissa with her family members, it's the family members who will become a sort of shared joke between Maggie and Melissa, one that helps the couple forge their own bond more securely.

A separation-individuation therapist would have some clear advice for Melissa, too. Melissa is not drinking a tremendous amount—not enough to affect her functioning—but she is definitely leaning on her nightly glasses of wine. And in separation-individuation theory, dependence is always a bad thing. Melissa's task is to grow strong enough that she doesn't need the wine. Or anything, or anyone, else.

At this point in the book, you might not see their problems in terms of the need to separate. You might see their problems differently. I certainly do. Right off the bat I notice that this relationship lacks sparkle. They're not bringing out the worst in each other—no one is uttering curses or breaking furniture—but they don't exactly come to life in each other's company, either. Trying desperately to feel better, Melissa has turned to wine. Maggie is hoping that a busy schedule, family time, and a whopping dose of television will produce good feelings.

These are classic signs of trouble with the Energetic pathway, which begins deep in your brain stem and travels a winding road until it ends in your orbitomedial prefrontal cortex, a part of your brain that helps you make decisions. Dopamine is a neurochemical that zips along this path and helps you feel simultaneously fulfilled and motivated. When dopamine is flowing, you don't feel like you've become a different person. That's what makes it so great. When you've got a steady supply of dopamine, you still feel like yourself, except that you feel like yourself on a really great day.

The human brain has evolved to get a burst of dopamine when it does something life-sustaining. Eating, drinking water, exercise, sex, and healthy relationships are all supposed to trigger feel-good sensations, to make us want to do the things that are good for us. But the brain loves to get dopamine, and if it can't get dopamine the ideal way, it will turn to other, less healthy, methods. Drugs and alcohol are common dopamine sources, but so are shopping, gaming, and obsessive eating. And, in Maggie's case, tight bonding with both one's family and one's television.

Problems that run along the Energetic pathway often look a lot like Maggie and Melissa's, in the sense that there is a basically loving relationship in which the fizziness has gone flat. I'm not speaking solely of romantic relationships here; dopamine is present in healthy friendships and family relationships, too. When the dopamine trickles out of one of those relationships, things don't feel fun anymore. You may try to accustom yourself to the drab, lackluster days. You may tell yourself that adult life isn't supposed to be fun. But eventually your brain will beg for some excitement. And, frankly, your brain is doing what it's built to do. It's telling you that it wants to claim its birthright; it wants to feel energized by its relationships. We are supposed to feel a sense of motivating satisfaction when we're with the people we love. Maybe not every minute, but most of the time. Moreover, we are capable of feeling that pop of good energy even in long-term relationships. In fact, our permanent relationships can be the most rewarding.

When a basically good relationship loses its sparkle, it's the Energetic pathway that is most obviously affected. Just look at Maggie and Melissa. Not only are they drinking and watching junk TV, they're so depleted they barely have the energy to snipe at each other. But often these Energetic symptoms are just the tip of the iceberg. To understand why the dopamine isn't flowing, you need to look at what's going on with *all* the C.A.R.E. pathways. Both women filled out the C.A.R.E. Relational Assessment, but I think you'll get a good sense of what was happening to them by looking at just Maggie's:

> **Here are Maggie's C.A.R.E. pathway scores:**
> **C**alm (add up scores for statements 1 through 7;
>   maximum total score is 175): **128 (moderate)**
> **A**ccepted (add up scores for statements 5 through 11;
>   maximum total score is 175): **144 (high)**
> **R**esonant (statements 12 through 16; maximum total
>   score is 125): **84 (moderate)**
> **E**nergetic (statements 17 through 20; maximum total
>   score is 100): **64 (moderate)**

Energy and Resonance: A Synergistic Pair

The Resonant and Energetic pathways tend to go up and down together—not always, but often. Maggie's low Resonant scores underscore what happens when your family doesn't want to see your full personality—and your partner can't see how much you need your family. No wonder she didn't feel so energetic. Imagine trying to squeeze good energy out of a relationship where you feel stifled. With these scores, Maggie is still highly functional, able to work and go

Maggie's C.A.R.E. Relational Assessment Chart

Answer the questions on a 1-to-5 scale: 1=None or never 2=Rarely or minimal 3=Some of the time 4=More often than not; medium high 5=Usually; very high	#1 Melissa	#2 Mom	#3 Jane (sister)	#4 Ken (brother)	#5 Karen (sister)	Total Statement Score	C.A.R.E. Code
1. I trust this person with my feelings.	4	3	4	4	3	18	Calm
2. This person trusts me with her feelings.	4	3	4	4	4	19	Calm
3. I feel safe being in conflict with this person.	3	3	3	3	3	15	Calm
4. This person treats me with respect.	4	4	4	4	3	19	Calm
5. In this relationship, I feel calm.	5	3	4	3	3	18	Calm Accepted
6. I can count on this person to help me out in an emergency.	4	5	5	4	4	22	Calm Accepted
7. In this relationship, it's safe to acknowledge our differences.	4	3	4	3	3	17	Calm Accepted
8. When I am with this person, I feel a sense of belonging.	5	5	5	5	5	25	Accepted
9. Despite our different roles, we treat each other as equals.	5	4	4	4	4	21	Accepted

Answer the questions on a 1-to-5 scale:	#1 Melissa	#2 Mom	#3 Jane (sister)	#4 Ken (brother)	#5 Karen (sister)	Total Statement Score	C.A.R.E. Code
10. I feel valued in this relationship.	4	5	5	4	4	**22**	Accepted
11. There is give and take in this relationship.	4	3	5	3	4	**19**	Accepted
12. This person is able to sense how I feel.	3	3	4	3	3	**16**	Resonant
13. I am able to sense how this person feels.	4	4	4	3	4	**19**	Resonant
14. With this person I have more clarity about who I am.	3	3	4	3	3	**16**	Resonant
15. I feel that we "get" each other.	3	3	4	4	3	**17**	Resonant
16. I am able to see that my feelings impact this person.	3	3	4	3	3	**16**	Resonant
17. This relationship helps me be more productive in my life.	4	3	3	3	3	**16**	Energetic
18. I enjoy the time I spend with this person.	3	3	4	3	3	**16**	Energetic
19. Laughter is a part of this relationship.	3	3	4	3	3	**16**	Energetic
20. In this relationship, I feel more energetic.	3	3	4	3	3	**16**	Energetic
Safety Group Score	**75**	**69**	**82**	**69**	**68**		

through the motions of the day. But don't most of us hope for more out of life than just going through the motions?

We agreed to try boosting their energy by attacking some of the resonance issues.

We also talked about how to see their marriage and their extended families in terms other than the "individuality versus sameness" debate. If Maggie wanted to feel good again, if she wanted to feel more emotional resonance with her family, she'd have to be her real self in front of her family and (this is the hard part) negotiate the awkwardness and conflict that would almost inevitably occur. Maggie's task would be to help her family see that her maturity was not a threat—it wasn't a sign of rejection, just a difference.

After several conversations about the best place to begin their efforts, Maggie and Melissa decided to take on the all-day Sundays at Maggie's parents' house. Maggie and Melissa decided that they would meet the family at church, but that they would go back to her mother's only once a month; they explained kindly to her family that this was one of the only days they got time alone, and they needed to spend it on their many projects and to simply catch up on their relationship.

If you can't imagine how an innocuous little announcement like this could have caused a problem, you've never lived in a family like Maggie's. Her mother immediately wondered aloud if Maggie and Melissa's marriage was in danger. Her sisters suggested that Maggie and Melissa were being snooty. Her brother felt generally angry and betrayed. For a couple of months, this new plan was the family's favored topic of conversation. Melissa felt embarrassed and excluded, and Maggie was surprised by the intensity of the pushback they'd received. But instead of returning to the either/or options that they once felt they had, they decided to ride out the discomfort. They stuck to their guns by staying away most Sundays—and they kept their promise by coming once a month. They showed the family that they were committed to being both independent and close. The time away allowed Maggie and Melissa to come to the gatherings once a month in a more refreshed state, in which they could be more appreciative of the group. It wasn't perfect. They missed the threads of many inside jokes, and for a while, they were mildly punished by being treated as outsiders. But after a while, everyone adjusted to the new normal. Miraculously, even Melissa started to enjoy visiting her in-laws.

You don't have to wait for relationship nirvana to get more dopamine, though. Early in the therapy process, I asked Maggie and Melissa to tell me about the beginning of their relationship. I often ask couples this question, and I do it for several reasons. When people first fall in love, their neural circuits are flooded with dopamine, in the same way that alcohol and drugs can flood the brain with dopamine. If the couple can revisit that blissful time together, they can wake up some of the good energy that's gone dormant. Maggie immediately remembered how thrilling it was to find someone like Melissa, so solid and well defined. So different from her family! At this point, both women started telling the story of their early relationship, sometimes finishing each other's sentences. It was as if they had transported back to a time when they could see each other clearly. Our goal, I told them, was to get that energy and clarity back into the relationship.

What if you can't remember the good times? This is a clue, telling you that the relationship is suffering from serious disconnection. You may still be able to plug back into each other, so if the relationship is important to you, please don't give up on it. For a few couples, the relationship has never gone through those initial heady days; these are usually relationships that were built around responsibility or guilt or some other compulsive feeling. These couples have a harder road ahead.

Ways to Reconnect the Dopamine Reward System to Healthy Relationships

Melissa and Maggie were enjoying each other more, but they found it difficult to give up their substitute sources of dopamine: wine and TV. I explained that during their year or two of crisis, their Energetic pathways had become rewired. Melissa's dopamine reward system was still connected to wine, Maggie's to TV. Now that they could feel some pleasure in their relationship again, it was an ideal time to step in and break this unwanted neural connection.

How Are You Stimulating Your Dopamine Reward System?

This exercise helps you get in touch with the primary ways you stimulate your dopamine pathways. You can pose the question like this:

How do I make myself feel better?

There is an endless number of things in the world that can supply dopamine, and that you can become addicted to. Here are some suggestions to get you thinking:

Relationships

Food

Drugs

Alcohol

Risk-taking activities

Shopping

Gambling

Sex

Working

Exercise

Internet surfing

Watching pornography

Check off any categories that apply to your life. If there are other behaviors that apply to you, add them. Then make a

rough assessment of what percentage of your feel-good time
is spent with each activity.

Source of Dopamine	Percentage of Feel-Good Time
Hanging out with my friends	10%
Shopping	20%
Exercising	15%
Eating	50%
Bungee jumping	5%

This exercise can unmask all sorts of interesting facts.
Like, hmmm, you often turn to food, sweets and carbohydrates particularly, when you need a lift. Exercise makes you
feel good but you don't do it that often. You don't call friends
when you're glum because you think that makes you "too
needy." Shopping always makes you feel better, at least until
you've spent too much money, and you run to the mall or shop
online more often than you realized. Bungee jumping is not a
frequent source of happiness, but you have done it a couple of
times and had to put it on the list because the euphoria afterward lifts your spirits for days.

When Rufus, the office worker who was addicted to Internet porn, did this exercise, he was shocked:

Source of Dopamine	Percentage of Feel-Good Time
Surfing porn sites	90%
Being with friends and family	5%
Ice cream	5%

As Rufus reflected on these results, he could easily see that over the course of the last few years he had become consumed with looking at pornography. His life had gotten very, very small.

For her part, Maggie's assessment helped her see she was spending more time with the TV than she'd realized. This unleashed some complicated feelings. For one thing, she didn't feel that the TV was "stupid." She described the relief she felt at the end of the day, when she'd jump into her pajamas, pour a cup of tea, and tune in to shows that were well-written dramas with intelligent character development. Some days, Maggie joked, she started to believe these characters were people in her actual life. In fact, this was Melissa's fear—that was she being elbowed aside by fictional people.

Identify Relationships That Are High in Zest

The next step is to identify your strongest sources of relational dopamine; these form your best shot at reconnecting your reward system. When Jean Baker Miller described growth-fostering relationships as producing a feeling of energy or zest, she was not thinking of dopamine. That zest is a palpable increase in energy, however, generated in part by elevated levels of dopamine, created by both of you. So go back to the C.A.R.E. Relational Assessment Chart and see which relationships produced the highest Energetic scores. Consciously stirring up good experiences with these people will exercise the neural circuitry between dopamine and rela-tionships, making the Energetic pathway stronger.

Rufus liked his guy friends, but in a placid, passive way. His most obvious source of relational zest was his sister. He thought she was sweet and kind and really cared about him. He asked her to dinner, and she was psyched; Rufus noticed that he felt a little lift in his chest when he realized she wanted to spend time with him. It was not the buzzing excitement and arousal of porn, but it was a sensation worth his atten-tion. The more time he could spend in relationships that cre-ated this feeling—and the more he paid attention to that feeling—the better. One day his friend Drew announced that he was getting married. Rufus was shocked: he thought that all his guy friends were bachelors for life. He found that he was curious to hear about Drew's experience with this woman, how excited and unembarrassed Drew was when he described her. Rufus felt a longing, halfway between his chest and belly, for a relationship with a real woman.

Melissa felt that drinking wine wasn't a big problem; it was a pleasant way to relax after a long, intense day at work. But she acknowledged that wine was taking focus and energy away from her relationships. She and Melissa agreed that two evenings a week, they'd make an extra effort to connect. Me-lissa suggested that they make dinner together and sit down to eat it without any distractions. This ended up being a pleasant and engaging way to spend time together. Melissa still had her glass of wine or even two, and sometimes Mag-gie joined her. On those evenings, drinking felt different—

not a way to numb out or escape, but simply a fun part of the meal.

Melissa also surprised herself by discovering that her parents—who were emotionally and physically distant— nevertheless scored high on her Energetic pathways. A few times a week, she called them at the end of the day. At first, they begged off the phone, saying that they knew she'd rather be with Maggie. Then, alarmed by the increased communication, they instructed Melissa to get off the phone and go take care of her marriage instead of calling them. But—and this is important—Melissa didn't let this awkwardness put her off. She kept up the phone calls, and kept asking questions about their lives, and as time went on, her parents were sharing funny stories about their day and their stresses at work. There were no big reveals, but there was enough connection to produce a nice shot of happiness.

Relabel and Refocus

Now it's time to make concrete change. First, recognize your habitual patterns. Do you turn to your addictions or bad habits when you have emotions that are uncomfortable? Twelve-step programs like Alcoholics Anonymous talk how about the urge to drink predictably comes on when you are hungry, angry, lonely, or tired. Those emotional and physical states form the acronym HALT, which perfectly describes what you should do when your feel the urge to participate in your bad habit. But in a culture that values logic over emotion, it can be hard to interpret what your body and mind are trying to tell you. If you have the urge to "use" something to feel better, try to pause and look inward to see if there is some emotion attached to the urge. For help identifying a full range of emotions, see pages 231–241.

If you're able to identify and label the feeling, see if you can watch it move by. Although a feeling can seem incredibly dangerous, it will not kill you. Feeling states are like the clouds; with time they simply dissipate.

If the feeling does not move on and your craving continues to be strong, relabel the craving. It's defeating to think of a troublesome habit as a failure of character or something that you just can't stop yourself from doing. Instead, label it for what it is: a neural pathway that's grown stronger with repeated use. I told Melissa that it would probably be too much for her to give up wine right away—her default neural pathways for wine were so strong that she would probably end up giving in. In a classic cycle, she'd feel bad about giving in . . . and then turn to more wine to help her feel better.

Instead, Melissa could say to herself, "Hmmm. I notice I really want to wind down with some wine. Okay. That's interesting. That neural pathway is *very* strong." Identifying the pathway for what it is—a series of neurons and not an inborn character flaw—is a first step toward releasing its hold over you. Recognize that whatever craving you have is just a desire to feel better, to get more dopamine. You can acknowledge that there are many other ways to stimulate dopamine that are healthier for you.

At this point, it's time to refocus your attention on one of those zestful relationships. Call up a positive relational moment with that person, one that is full of joy and humor—the more good energy, the better. (For an explanation of PRMs, see page 157.) If you're in a romantic relationship that's lost its energy, try mining your earliest days together. Chances are you'll find moments that are rich in dopamine.

If you feel comfortable, you could invite one or two of these people to participate in the refocusing process with you. They may have some dopamine-stimulating strategies they'd like to change, too. Agree that when you have a craving, you'll reach out to each other. If you can meet in person, great: you'll have the complete physiology of connection working for you and against the self-destructive craving. But if that's not possible, a phone call or text will help to break the immediate craving and ground you in healthier coping strategies.

I asked Rufus if he would call his sister in the evenings, just to catch up on the day, and see if that helped dislodge his habit a little. He disliked the idea but tried it twice—and on one of those two evenings, he found that calling his sister helped him avoid porn. He wondered aloud if this was cheating, because it wasn't the quality of the conversation that helped him; rather, he thought it was creepy to watch porn after speaking with his little sister.

"I'll take that," I said. "Talking to your sister allows you to pause and think." Rufus wasn't cheating. It was the brainless drifting to porn that was so problematic for him. When he could interrupt that drifting, it was possible for him to make better choices . . . including reconnecting healthy relationships to his dopamine reward system.

By lifting your thoughts up out of their well-worn neural track and moving them toward a healthy relationship, you're putting all three rules of brain change in motion. And by pairing your neural pathway for craving dopamine with your neural pathway for feeling connected to a friend, you'll eventually wire those two pathways back together. You'll begin to crave relationship, not wine or ice cream or even bungee jumping, when you want a lift.

Starve Neural Pathways That Say, "You Should Learn to Feel Better on Your Own"

How many times have you been encouraged to self-regulate your emotions, deal with pain on your own, work out your troubles independently? This strategy is endemic in societies that see separation as a sign of maturity. This value is stored in your mind and in every cell in your body, so that when you are hungry, angry, lonely, or tired you learn that you are to take care of those needs on your own. That's what adults do! In fact, if you regularly turn to others for comfort, you can be called *codependent*. A whole self-help industry has built up around battling codependence in people—mostly women.

The truth, though, is that when humans successfully manage their emotions, they *never* do it alone. In fact, being completely alone is so toxic to the human brain and body that in most prison systems the last-ditch disciplinary tool is solitary confinement. If our brains were truly meant to self-regulate, solitary confinement would be a piece of cake and a pleasure. Instead, it's considered radical punishment and, according to some, a form of torture.

The goal of this exercise is the opposite of self-regulation. It's to learn how to regulate your emotions within growth-fostering relationships. Give this one some time; this is perhaps the most difficult relational skill to master when you've been steeped in a world that undermines relationships. Mutual regulation means that you and another person are invested and engaged in your growth and development. As we mutually grow, we each develop rich positive relational images tied to our pathways for connection—deep, strong body and mind memories stored in our cells of what human connection feels like. Intentionally or not, we refer to these images constantly to help us manage our stress levels. They're like a soft blanket to protect our psyches.

We'll call again on the first rule of brain change: **Use it or lose it.** Neural pathways compete for brain space, so if you want these good relational images to flourish, you must starve the pathways that are vying for real estate in your head. These are the pathways that carry the social messages that it is better to do things on your own, or that you are weak if you turn to others with your sadness or anger. Spend an afternoon or a day watching how often these messages float through your brain. Whenever you catch one, simply relabel it as a cultural message that sabotages your goal of reclaiming your connected brain. Immediately move your mind to a PRM, or to a stored image of a time you were supported and how good that felt. With practice, the world can transform in front of your eyes from one filled with competitors to one filled with helpers.

With this step, you've reached the end of the C.A.R.E. program. People who take the C.A.R.E. workshops often comment that the program works directly on the relational issues that have troubled them the most. For all its transparency, they say that the C.A.R.E. program is also rich, textured, and surprising—just like the best relationships. As you continue to grow within your relationships, a word of caution: whatever struggles you encounter, don't judge yourself harshly. Judging yourself will only throw your sympathetic nervous system into hyperdrive, making it harder for you to create the kind of change you're looking for.

As I see it, the C.A.R.E. program is a bridge that leads from isolation to connection. Exactly how far that bridge extends is up to you. Does the bridge arc toward a better relationship with your spouse? Your entire family? Your workplace, neighborhood, or community? Once you experience relationships that feel Calmer, more Accepting, Resonant, Energetic, and you may be surprised at how far you decide to travel.

Chapter 9

MAINTAIN YOUR BRAIN

As I write this chapter, there is a trend toward reality TV shows featuring people who demonstrate how to survive by yourself in the wild. You can learn some pretty interesting things from these shows: how to make a meal from frozen yak eyeballs, and how to use your pants as a flotation device. Most of all, the hosts impress on us, is the importance of physical fitness and adaptability. You've got to be able to leap over boulders. You've got to be strong enough to build a snow cave. Sometimes you'll have to run from wild pigs.

I love these shows. They're fun. But I can also see that the trend toward survival TV reflects our attitudes about separation, that surviving on your own is the truest, most elemental human situation, and the ultimate test of your maturity. Physical survival is an extension of how we see the social waters:

menacing, competitive, best navigated with a knife clenched between your teeth and a wary eye out for crocodiles.

Throughout this book I've tried to demonstrate an alternate way of thinking about our capacity for psychological maturity and growth. How our brains are designed to use relationships to help them grow and stretch and change. How those same brains contain neural pathways that can flourish only when given input from healthy relationships. How we mature, not by stepping away from other people but by moving into greater relational complexity. So maybe it won't be surprising that I'm offering a different way to think of fitness as well. I want you to begin thinking about a brain that is physically fit—a brain that, like a survivalist's body, can remain strong and flexible, and can adapt to changing conditions. Maybe not the conditions of an active volcano in a Pacific archipelago, but the relational terrain that changes as you meet new people, as technology creates different ways of interacting, as your own growth changes the nature of your relationships. At the beginning of this book, I compared relationships to a magician's interlocking rings. The acts of coming together, overlapping, moving away, and integrating what you've learned, require you to stay light on your feet, mentally speaking. For this, your brain needs relationships—but it also needs to stay physically fit. It needs to conduct electrical impulses with efficiency. It needs to grow new blood vessels and neurons. It needs to rest and recover.

Below are nine ways to keep your brain in shape for great relationships.

274 FOUR WAYS TO CLICK

1. Drink Water.

At my neighborhood pool, there is a rule that if you hear thunder or see lightning, everyone must immediately get out of the water and remain out for thirty minutes. Every summer, the neighborhood children complain that their happy pool time is interrupted for what to them appears to be no good reason. They don't realize that this rule is lifesaving. The free ions, salts, and other minerals and metals that are found in water are highly efficient conductors of electricity. If lightning hits the water, its current travels almost instantaneously through the pool.

The same principle operates in your brain, which uses electrical currents to send its signals from one nerve to another. These signals include the impulses that zip from neuron to neuron along the smart vagus and eventually to the sympathetic and parasympathetic nervous systems, sending your autonomic nervous system accurate data about whether to stand up and fight or sit down and relax. Signals along the mirroring system let you have the imitative responses that produce an almost instant reading of another person. To do this and other complex, fast relational computation, your neurons need to be plump and well hydrated.

The Institute of Medicine of the National Academy of Sciences recommends that women have a total intake of 91 ounces of water per day; men should get 125 ounces daily. We get about 20 percent of these water needs through food, however, and most of us will do just fine by drinking whenever we're thirsty, or by drinking enough to produce clear or pale yellow urine. Caffeine and alcohol are diuretics, so if you consume these, you'll need to drink extra water to compensate. Also drink extra water if you exercise for more than an hour in a day.

2. Exercise Your Brain as Well as Your Body.

If you currently exercise to improve your stamina, shape your body, or save your heart, you are already ahead in the brain game. It's been known for a while that exercise gives you the so-called runner's high by increasing your endorphins, the natural morphine produced in your brain. But exercise does far more. Regular exercise increases key neurotransmitters like serotonin, dopamine, and norepinephrine, all of which support your mood and energy level. It also increases a recently discovered neurochemical called *brain-derived neurotrophic factor,* or BDNF, which improves your rate of learning. In his book *Spark: The Revolutionary New Science of Exercise and the Brain,* John Ratey, a clinical professor of psychiatry at Harvard Medical School, documents a novel physical education program called Zero Hour. Created in the Naperville, Illinois, school system seventeen years ago, Zero Hour has kids perform aerobic exercise at 80 to 90 percent of their maximum heart rate before the day's classes begin. The

effects on learning have been dramatic. The district consistently ranks in the state's top ten for academics, despite
spending significantly less per student than the state's other
top-performing districts. One reason for these results could
be that there is more electrical activity in the brains of fit
children than in sedentary kids. Another is BDNF. Ratey
writes, "BDNF gives the synapses the tools they need to take
in information, process it, remember it, and put it in context."[1]
Exercise also increases an important chemical, *vascular endothelial growth factor,* that supports the growth of blood vessels
in organs and tissues throughout your body and brain. More
blood vessels means more blood flow and more blood flow
means more oxygen and nutrients sent to your brain cells. In
Ratey's words, "exercise prepares neurons to connect, while
mental stimulation allows your brain to capitalize on that
readiness."[2]

To stimulate neurotransmitters, BDNF, and vascular
endothelial growth factor—and to sharpen mental acuity in
general—it is better to partake of cardiovascular exercise
than to lift weights or do yoga. It appears that the crucial
factor is getting your heart rate up and keeping it there. Ratey
suggests performing cardiovascular exercise at these levels:

Two days each week, exercise at 70 to 75 percent of your
maximum heart rate (so that you are sweaty and somewhat
breathless) for 30 to 60 minutes; *and*

Four days each week, exercise at 60 to 65 percent of your
max heart rate (you're still sweaty at this level, but you can
talk fairly easily) for 30 to 60 minutes.[3]

I know. It's a lot of exercise, more than the amount recommended by the Centers for Disease Control to maintain physical health. If you struggle to get going, leverage the benefits of human interaction. A Stanford University study found that when people received a phone call about their workouts every two weeks, subjects increased their exercise amounts by 78 percent.[4] And the department of kinesiology at Indiana University discovered that couples who worked out separately had a 43 percent dropout rate in an exercise program, while only about 7 percent of couples who exercised together dropped out.[5] Remember that relational dopamine is a great way to melt old neural pathways and create ones that lead to new, better habits.

3. Get Omega-3 Fatty Acids Through Food or Supplements.

Some people call the brain "gray matter," but if you look at a picture of your brain, you'll see that it actually looks whitish. The source of that white color is fat—and a fatty brain is a very good thing, because it speeds the transmission of electrical signals. Omega-3 fatty acids in particular are an essential component of cell membranes. They also help replace damaged brain cells by promoting the growth of new neurons, and they may be protective against anxiety and mood disorders.[6]

There are three types of omega-3 fatty acids: EPA, DHA,

and ALA. While all three are good for your body, only EPA and DHA can cross the blood–brain barrier and nourish your brain cells. Perhaps the easiest way to get EPA or DHA is from natural sources such as salmon, herring, or tuna. Eating these fish two or three times per week will boost your brain functioning. For the non-fish-eater, taking a daily supplement of EPA or DHA is a great alternative and can be found in most local pharmacies and grocery stores.

You'll also need antioxidants. When your body metabolizes fatty acids, the by-products include free radicals, which can build up and disrupt protein and lipid development—and damage your DNA. The buildup of free radicals is referred to as having a high load of *oxidative stress*. Antioxidants like vitamins C and E can bind to the free radicals and lower this stress. It's best to get your antioxidants from brightly colored fruits and vegetables, but you can also take a supplement if necessary.

4. Wear a Helmet When Putting Your Brain at Risk.

Daniel Amen, a psychiatrist who has pioneered the use of brain imaging with single photon emission computed tomography (SPECT) to help diagnose and treat mental illness and brain injury, describes the texture of the human brain as similar to medium-firm tofu. If you have ever cooked with tofu, you will realize that this comparison is *not* reassuring. Even though this tofu sits within the hard human skull, the skull has a number of peaks and valleys that form sharp edges. When your head is hit with something—whether a soccer ball or the windshield of a car—and the tofu is jostled within the skull even a small amount, it can sustain significant injuries. The resulting brain bruise, usually referred to as a *concussion*, can have detrimental effects months and even years after the initial injury.

As a mom and a psychiatrist, I am thrilled that my son did not want to play football, a game that puts your brain at risk during every play. Additionally, I frown on bouncing the ball off the front part of the skull in soccer. The prefrontal cortex is simply too precious and too important in regulating executive functioning and impulse control to have it hit over and over again. For this same reason, I recommend helmets for anyone participating in contact sports; motorcycle and bicycle riding; skateboarding, skiing, and snowboarding; and under any condition where it is possible for you to bang your head.

5. Spend Time in the Sun.

One of the easiest things you can do for your brain is to spend time in the sun. The sun's rays don't simply bounce off your skin (or fry it). They actually have an integral role in supporting your health. Those long summer days we all look forward to after a dark winter actually improve blood flow in your brain and help regulate key neurotransmitters, serotonin and melatonin. Serotonin helps to maintain a positive mood and a focused, calm outlook on life. It's also a precursor to melatonin, which—aside from physical benefits like helping the body counter infection, inflammation, autoimmune responses, and even cancer—assists with the onset of sleep. Sleep, as you'll see in a moment, is critical to healthy brain functioning. Sunlight also increases vitamin D levels, which affect both your mood and memory.

In the sun-crazy days of my youth, people set up tinfoil boxes and slathered themselves with oil in an effort to bake themselves like potatoes in an oven. This practice ignored one of the eternal rules of health—moderation—and decades later, these men and women were developing skin cancers at an alarming rate. Suntan lotions and oils were developed to filter some of the more aggressive sun rays and protect the skin; then sunscreens gave way to sunblocks that can offer more than one hundred times your natural protection against the sun. Now we have a generation of people who aren't getting enough sun, and who suffer from low levels of vitamin D. Once again, it all goes back to moderation. Try to get a little sunshine every day if you can. If you live in an area where that's not possible, the recommended dose for people without a clear vitamin D deficiency is 600 to 800 IUs daily. People with a vitamin D deficiency should supplement with 2,000 units a day until the deficiency has been remedied. Your doctor should evaluate your blood levels of vitamin D during your regular checkup.

6. Get Enough Sleep.

Like getting an adequate amount of sunlight, getting enough sleep is a freebie—sort of. It's awfully easy to stay up an extra hour to watch a show because, finally, the kids are asleep and this is "your" time. When I was in medical school, there was a clear improvement in status for the person who could stay awake the longest and still perform on a high level. I have vivid memories (or maybe flashbacks) of spending nights in the emergency room seeing patient after patient and guzzling Diet Coke after Diet Coke to stay awake.

Yet even small amounts of sleep deprivation can cause multiple problems in the brain and body, including poor concentration, drowsiness, impaired memory, impaired physical performance, a decrease in ability to do math calculations, and mood swings. "Your time" at the end of the night is much better spent sleeping. You might notice that when you actually get enough sleep, you have more energy and focus to get through the list of things in the day that are usually left to the end. Research also shows that even though you might get used to functioning with a sleep debt, your reaction time and judgment can still be significantly impaired. That's because less sleep will create more irritable brain pathways.

Sleep needs depend on your age and, of course, on your own specific brain and body, but in general, adults need seven to eight hours of sleep a night (though a few people need as little as five or as much as ten), teenagers need roughly nine hours of sleep, and infants need a whopping sixteen hours of sleep per day. Remember, too little sleep creates a sleep debt that eventually has to be repaid!

7. Eat Brain Foods.

There is a connection between your gastrointestinal tract and your nervous system, and what you eat has a major impact on how your brain functions. The proteins, carbohydrates, and fats you eat become the building blocks for cells and neurotransmitters in your brain. Micronutrients, like vitamins and cofactors, are needed to run the little factories in your cells and produce energy. A balanced diet, including all of the essential food groups and plenty of fruits and vegetables, will make your body healthier and your brain work more efficiently.

But you can and should go beyond the traditional balanced diet when you're focusing on brain health. The brain foods listed here have specific benefits to mental and psychological functioning. Blueberries help prevent oxidative stress; in rats, they've been shown to enhance learning. Avocados and whole grains help preserve blood flow to the entire brain, including its C.A.R.E. pathways. Beans deliver a regular stream of glucose to the brain, providing a steady (not wild or erratic) supply of energy. Freshly brewed tea is an ideal drink, because it contains the ideal amount of caffeine to improve focus, mood, and memory. Tea also contains small amounts of catechin, which helps regulate blood flow. Nuts and seeds contain vitamin E, which helps stave off cognitive decline. Dark chocolate pulls off a hat trick with endorphins to calm the body and brain, caffeine for focus, and antioxidants to fight free radicals. The final brain food is any fish that contains the omega-3 fatty acids I've talked about: wild salmon, herring, and tuna.

8. Use a Brain Training Program.

Most of us know to keep our brains stimulated with games and activities, but not all stimulation expands overall brain functioning. If you are routinely doing crossword puzzles to keep your brain alive and active, it is likely that what is increasing for you is . . . your capacity to do crossword puzzles. Posit Science, a company founded by neuroscientist Michael Merzenich, has designed the SAAGE protocol to describe the benefits that brain games should include:

S is for *speed*. As your brain ages, the speed of
   electrical transmission slows. A good brain activity
   should improve the speed of your thinking.
A is for *accuracy*. Brain games should improve how
   well you classify pieces of information.
A is for *adaptivity*. Brain games need to adapt to your
   specific and current level of functioning. If you are
   having an off day, the tasks should get a little

easier. The last thing your brain needs is to play a game at which you are constantly failing; it's not helpful for your C.A.R.E. pathways or your learning to stimulate the sympathetic nervous system unnecessarily.

G stands for *generalizability*, which refers to the ability for the program to improve real-life activities, not just the activity in the game (e.g., crossword puzzles).

E is for *engagement*. For adults to turn on their learning machinery, the nucleus basalis, novelty and attention are required; the reward system stimulates dopamine to help solidify new pathways. A game should engage the brain's attention, reward, and novelty systems hundreds of times per training hour. These systems must be engaged for long-lasting brain change.[7]

For a list of brain-change programs that fit all the SAAGE requirements, visit www.sharpbrains.com.

9. Find Stress-Reduction Techniques You Love.

Stress, and the stress chemicals it produces, can be remarkably toxic to your brain. But like most things in your body, there is a continuum of toxicity. Studies have shown that at mild levels, stress can actually help you improve your cognitive capacity. The release of adrenaline wakes up nerve pathways, allowing you to focus and concentrate better. As the stress level increases, however, the system turns on you—and the same chemicals that just a minute ago allowed you to focus more closely now cause you to feel anxious and panicky.

From an evolutionary perspective, the system makes sense. Imagine you are a caveperson, scanning the environment for danger. Being just stressed enough to stay alert and avoid spacing out is crucial to your survival. Off in the distance, you see a mountain lion on the prowl. The adrenaline simmers in your body and you remain attentive, but not reactive. After ten minutes, you notice the mountain lion seems to be stalking closer and closer to your cave. More adrenaline pumps through your nervous system and now your heart is starting to beat faster, your breaths are becoming shorter, your body is making the switch from scanning and evaluation to preparation for battle. If you are a cavewoman, a combination of adrenaline and the hormone oxytocin gives you the energy, focus, and wisdom to gather the other members of the clan and their children into a protective huddle. If you are a caveman, your testosterone and vasopressin rise, and you are thinking of tearing the mountain lion apart in order to defend your tribe.

Your stress response can be your friend and ally, helping you navigate a complicated and occasionally dangerous world.

However, when we socialize humans to be autonomous and not turn to others to help buffer stress, we actively undermine the development of the neural pathways for connection. These neural pathways are an essential balance to the sympathetic nervous system and help keep it in check so that you are not in a state of high arousal all the time.

People who develop post-traumatic stress disorder from childhood abuse, domestic violence, or war live with a sympathetic nervous system that is running full blast much of the time, and this response is incredibly destructive. The cortisol released in an effort to counter the high levels of adrenaline can be toxic to the hippocampus, the area of the brain that stores memories. It can also help create a cascade of physical destruction, leading to the development of chronic health problems, from diabetes to autoimmune disorders. And of course, having an overactive stress response system makes it even harder to build healthy relationships.

For all these reasons, if you are spending much of your life in a culture that actively cuts off your C.A.R.E. pathways, it is essential that you balance the excessive stress response with some activity that reduces stress. Start by simply focusing on your breath throughout the day. When you are stressed, your breathing becomes more superficial and rapid, which leads to less oxygen to your brain . . . which can lead to more irritable neurons and ultimately more stress. So throughout the day, pause every now and then and focus on taking ten deep breaths. You will quickly feel the impact of increased oxygen to your brain. The beauty of this technique is that you can do

it anytime, on the subway or at your desk, even in an annoying meeting with a colleague—and no one will notice.

Anything that reduces your stress can be a stress-
reduction activity; on page 163, you'll find a list of suggestions
for soothing a jumpy sympathetic nervous system. These are
tried-and-true stress busters. The important thing is for you
to pick something you can commit to, because balancing your
autonomic nervous system is like everything else you are trying to change in your brain: it takes practice. Many people
use meditation, yoga, and other forms of mindfulness, but
if these aren't for you, think of what does decrease your stress.
If playing with your children at the end of the day allows you
to feel safe and out of the stressful world, then build this activity into your day. If going for a run at lunch allows you
to dispel the neurochemicals of distress, then make time for
it. The goal is to counteract the ongoing stress that comes
from spending much of your time in a culture that undermines your primary way to reduce stress: growth-fostering
relationships.

C.A.R.E. FOR LIFE

As I've just noted, balancing your autonomic nervous system
takes practice. So does strengthening all four of your C.A.R.E.
pathways. Not only does it take practice to heal your connected brain, it *is* a practice, in the same sense that yoga or
meditation is a practice. At first, learning to nourish your
neural pathways for feeling Calm, Accepted, Resonant, and

Energetic will feel awkward. It may feel as if you're work-ing against everything your culture has taught you about relationships—and, in fact, that's exactly what you're doing. But work on the C.A.R.E. pathways often enough and they will thrive. Soon, growing and sustaining healthy relation-ships will feel more natural.

It is time to send parents a new instruction manual for raising their children; it is time to send our children a new set of rules for interacting with friends and enemies; it is time to make our business leaders a new template for helping employ-ees work cooperatively; and it is time to teach our world lead-ers how to guide their communities to fulfill their capacities to connect. We need an approach to human relationships that accurately reflects how interconnected we all are and nour-ishes our ability to use healthy relationships for richer, health-ier lives.

It's often said that a culture changes one person at a time, and that the only person you can change is yourself. But when you realize that we are not separated by strict boundaries, and that our relationships have a neurological life that unfolds inside the brains and minds of everyone we encounter, those statements seem too limiting. The minute you make a change in the way you relate to people—when you become less judg-mental, more curious, less fearful, more accepting—you also make a shift in the places where you and other people overlap. When you improve your pathways for connection, the artifi-cial walls that support the separation mentality melt away;

those boundaries transform into rich areas of human interface, abuzz with growth and energy.

In other words, when a relationship changes, it quite literally changes the minds of everyone in that relationship. Your
own transformation isn't limited to yourself alone, because
you are not alone. We live within one another.

ACKNOWLEDGMENTS

I have heard authors say, "It takes a village to write a book," but if you have Leigh Ann Hirschman on your team, you can do it with a small neighborhood. Leigh Ann and I took a leap of faith in writing a book that challenges the deep-seated cultural belief in autonomy. It was a leap best done in tandem. Leigh Ann wore many hats—beginning as a consultant and wise editor, shifting to the role of brilliant writer, and ending as a trusted friend. Her integrity, good humor, and attention to detail far surpassed my expectations. By the end of the project, Leigh Ann had clarified and accentuated my thoughts and ideas, saying what I wanted to say far better than I could have said it. Thank you, Leigh Ann.

I am grateful to my agents, Kathryn Beaumont and Katherine Flynn from Kneerim, Williams & Bloom, who believed in this book and helped it find both a home and an enthusiastic editor, Sara Carder at Tarcher.

Christina Robb was instrumental in birthing this book.

As my writing coach, she gently read early drafts of the manuscript and convinced me that every writer struggles to find her voice. When I coughed up a twenty-page hairball, she calmly and kindly pointed out that I was clearing my throat for the first fifteen pages.

Mike Miller has been relentless in his support for the work done at the Jean Baker Miller Training Institute. His message has been clear and consistent: take yourselves seriously, write books, and promote the message of the centrality of relationships to health and well-being. Mike's ongoing support and culturally relevant clippings that arrive by snail mail continue to remind me there is a broader context to this work.

Roseann Adams, a friend and colleague, used the early C.A.R.E. Relational Assessment with her clients and provided me with invaluable feedback on the structure and impact of the tool. Through the years, I have gotten both support and helpful feedback from generous participants attending our annual intensive summer institute. This community of relational-cultural practitioners remains central to the creation and dissemination of the work associated with JBMTI. I am especially appreciative of Dr. Constance Gunderson and her colleagues at St. Scholastica, who are working with me on a research project focused on the effectiveness of the C.A.R.E. program in social work students. Mary Vicario has been exceedingly clever at taking relational neuroscience and creating activities for parents and children. Her enthusiasm for the work is contagious.

I have had the privilege of working with and learning from my two friends and colleagues at JBMTI, Maureen Walker and Judith Jordan. Maureen has the mind of a scholar, the heart of an activist, and the soul of a theologian. Listening to Maureen is a religious experience. Her thoughts and ideas have shaped my thinking and writing on the cultural context of relationships. Judith Jordan's prolific writings, intense intellectual curiosity, and Buddhist energy infuse relational-cultural theory (or RCT) with heart and soul.

Dan Siegel's work on the neurobiology of relationships continues to shape my own. His support for this project and endorsement of my work are deeply appreciated. It has been a pleasure becoming a "mwe" ("me" plus "we") with him.

I spend most of my days connecting with clients in my private practice. It is not always easy, but it is always interesting. In each of these relationships, I have grown, and I feel lucky that so many have trusted me with their most intimate feelings and life experiences.

My life and neural pathways have been deeply shaped by Melissa Coco, Angel Seibring, and Frank Anderson, who have supported the creation of this book directly and indirectly by reading early drafts and by providing friendship and distraction when I needed to recharge. I am indebted to Pamela Peck, a supervisor and friend who introduced me to RCT early in my residency. I clicked with the theory immediately, and it has been a guiding light in my personal and professional life.

For the past twenty-five years, I have been working with

Cindy Kettyle to reshape my own relational templates. Although she knows I hate that psychoanalytic couch in her home office (it looks like she dragged it from Vienna), Cindy has been the perfect therapist and confidant for me. In this relationship, I have laughed my way to health.

The revolutionary and courageous work of Jean Baker Miller, Irene Stiver, Judith Jordan, and Jan Surrey, who were the founding scholars at the Stone Center (which eventually was called the Jean Baker Miller Training Institute). They paved the way for my generation of clinicians and scholars to promote connection with very little shame. Their prophetic theory feeds a movement that continues to reshape Western culture.

My brother, Philip Banks, is the only person I know who could learn an entire computer language in one evening. Your love and support is greatly appreciated.

My older sister, Kate Banks, is a writer and healer who has been a role model for me in following the path less traveled, no matter where it has taken me.

My younger sister, Nancy Banks, is a fellow teacher and cultural critic. Her presence in my life has been equal parts love and laughter.

Finally, my deceased parents, Dr. Ronald F. Banks and Helena Poland Banks, both educators, gave me two invaluable gifts: the appreciation of teaching and learning, and the acceptance of my quirky differences.

NOTES

CHAPTER 1: BOUNDARIES ARE OVERRATED: A NEW WAY OF LOOKING AT RELATIONSHIPS

1 Giacomo Rizzolatti, Luciano Fadiga, Vittorio Gallese, and Leonardo Fogassi, "Premotor Cortex and the Recognition of Motor Actions," *Cognitive Brain Research* 3 (1996): 131–41.

2 Lea Winerman, "The Mind's Mirror," *Monitor on Psychology* 36, no. 9 (2005): 48.

3 Marco Iacoboni, *Mirroring People: The New Science of How We Connect with Others* (New York: Farrar, Straus, and Giroux, 2008), 267.

4 Judith Jordan, in discussion with the author, May 2014.

5 Sigmund Freud, *Beyond the Pleasure Principle*, The International Psycho-Analytic Library (London: The International Psychoanalytical Press, 1922), chapter IV.

6 D. G. Blazer, "Social Support and Mortality in an Elderly Community Population," *American Journal of Epidemiology* 155, no. 5 (1982): 684–94.

7 T. E. Seeman and S. L. Syme, "Social Networks and Coronary Artery Disease: A Comparison of Structure and Function of Social Relations as Predictors of Disease," *Psychosomatic Medicine* 49, no. 4 (1987): 341–54.

8 P. L. Graves, C. B. Thomas, and L. A. Mead, "Familial and

Psychological Predictors of Cancer," *Cancer Detection & Prevention* 15, no. 1 (1991): 59–64.

9 L. G. Russek and G. E. Schwartz, "Narrative Descriptions of Parental Love and Caring Predict Health Status in Midlife: A 35-Year Follow-up of the Harvard Mastery of Stress Study," *Alternative Therapies in Health and Medicine* 2 (1996): 55–62.

CHAPTER 2: THE FOUR NEURAL PATHWAYS
FOR HEALTHY RELATIONSHIPS

1 N. I. Eisenberger and M. Lieberman, "Why It Hurts to Be Left Out: The Neurocognitive Overlap between Physical and Social Pain," in K. D. Williams, J. P. Forgas, and W. von Hippel (eds.), *The Social Outcast: Ostracism, Social Exclusion, Rejection, and Bullying* (New York: Cambridge University Press, 2005), 109–27.

2 P. M. Niedenthal, L. W. Barsalou, P. Winkielman, S. Krauth-Gruber, and F. Ric, "Embodiment in Attitudes, Social Perception, and Emotion," *Personality and Social Psychology Review* 9 (2005): 184–211.

3 S. M. Wilson, A. P. Saygin, M. I. Sereno, and M. Iacoboni, "Listening to Speech Activates Motor Areas Involved in Speech Production," *Nature Neuroscience* 7 (2004): 701–702.

4 I. Meister, S. M. Wilson, C. Deblieck, A. D. Wu, and M. Iacoboni, "The Essential Role of Premotor Cortex in Speech Perception," *Current Biology* 17 (2007): 1692–96.

5 D. Neal and T. Chartrand, "Embodied Emotion Perception, Amplifying and Dampening Facial Feedback Modulates Emotion Perception Accuracy," *Social Psychological and Personality Science* 2, no. 6 (2011): 673–78.

6 Diana Martinez, Daria Orlowska, Rajesh Narendran, Mark Slifstein, Fei Liu, Dileep Kumar, Allegra Broft, Ronald Van Heertum, and Herbert D. Kleber, "Dopamine Type 2/3 Receptor Availability in the Striatum and Social Status in Human Volunteers," *Biological Psychiatry* 67, no. 3 (2010): 275–78.

7 Louis Cozolino, *The Neuroscience of Human Relationships* (New York: W. W. Norton, 2014).

CHAPTER 3: THE THREE RULES OF BRAIN CHANGE

1   Antonio M. Battro, *Half a Brain Is Enough: The Story of Nico* (Cambridge, Mass.: Cambridge University Press, 2001).
2   Norman Doidge, *The Brain That Changes Itself* (New York: Penguin, 2006).
3   Martha Burns, "Dopamine and Learning: What the Brain's Reward System Can Teach Educators," *Scientific Learning*, http://www.scilearn.com/blog/dopamine-learning-brains-reward-center-teach-educators.php#.U3LnkwjDs3s.gmail (accessed May 13, 2014).

CHAPTER 5: C IS FOR CALM:
MAKE YOUR SMART VAGUS SMARTER

1   Jeffrey Schwartz, *Brain Lock: Free Yourself from Obsessive-Compulsive Behavior* (New York: Harper Perennial, 1997).

CHAPTER 7: R IS FOR RESONANT:
STRENGTHEN YOUR BRAIN'S MIRRORING SYSTEM

1   Cozolino, *The Neuroscience of Human Relationships*, 202.
2   Iacoboni, *Mirroring People*, 204–209.

CHAPTER 9: MAINTAIN YOUR BRAIN

1   John Ratey, *Spark: The Revolutionary New Science of Exercise and the Brain* (New York: Little, Brown, 2008), 45.
2   Ibid., 207.
3   Ibid., 242.
4   A. C. King, R. Friedman, B. Marcus, C. Castro, M. Napolitano, D. Alm, and L. Baker, "Ongoing Physical Activity Advice by Humans versus Computers: The Community Health Advice by Telephone (CHAT) Trial," *Health Psychology* 26, no. 6 (2007): 718–27.
5   J. P. Wallace, J. S. Raglin, and C. A. Jastremski, "Twelve Month Adherence of Adults Who Joined a Fitness Program with a Spouse vs. Without a Spouse," *Journal of Sports Medicine and Physical Fitness* 35, no. 3 (1995): 206–13.
6   Stuart Wolpert, "Scientists Learn How What You Eat Affects

Your Brain—And Those of Your Kids," *UCLA Newsroom*, http://newsroom.ucla.edu/releases/scientists-learn-how-food-affects-52668 (accessed May 14, 2014).

7   Posit Science, "Company FAQ," http://www.brainhq.com/about/company-faq (accessed May 14, 2014).

INDEX

Page numbers in **bold** indicate charts.

secrets, Accepted, 203–5
self-control approach, 67–68
self-help industry, 269
self-regulation (starving), Energetic,
    269–71
sensory neurons, 5
separation-individuation theory, 8–10,
    11, 13–14, 24, 44, 47, 55, 59–60,
    62, 67, 252–54, 272–73
serotonin, 37, 80, 275, 279–80
serotonin reuptake inhibitors (SSRIs),
    154
sharpbrains.com, 284
Siegel, Daniel J., ix–x
signs that a relationship supports
    Accepted pathway, 173
    Calm pathway, 135
    Energetic pathway, 248
    Resonant pathway, 208
Sinatra, Frank, 201
single photon emission computed
    tomography (SPECT),
    278
sleep importance, 280, 281–82
smart vagus nerve, 19–20, 31–32,
    33–35, 38–40, 139–41
    See also Calm: The Smart Vagus
social disconnection, 40–42, 43–48, 62,
    194
social pain overlap theory (SPOT),
    Accepted, 20, 178, 195–202
somatosensory cortex, 6, 54, 209
sorting your relationships into safety
    groups (C.A.R.E. Relational
    Assessment step three), 89, 90,
    98–101
*Spark: The Revolutionary New Science of
    Exercise and the Brain* (Ratey),
    275–76
speaking and listening connection, 49,
    50
Speed, Accuracy, Adaptivity,
    Generalizability, Engagement
    (SAAGE), 283–84
spending more time in resonant
    relationships, 221–24, **222**
Stanford University, 277

starving
    neural pathways that separate
        feelings from thoughts,
        Resonant, 231–33
    parasympathetic nervous system,
        Calm, 150, 170–72
    sympathetic nervous system, Calm,
        150–64
    unwanted relational images,
        Resonant, 245–47
    "you should learn to feel better on
        your own," Energetic,
        269–71
Stiver, Irene, 9
stress-reduction and brain, 284–87
stress response, near-constant
    activation of, 38–40
striatum, 59
Stryker, Rod, 163
sunlight and brain, 279–80, 281
super mirroring system, Resonant,
    52–53, 54
surprise, 224, 228
Surrey, Janet, 9, 168, 169
survival TV, 272–73
sympathetic nervous system
    danger, 30, 31, 32, 33–34, 35, 36–37,
        38, 39, 103, 139, 149, 150
    starving, Calm, 150–64
synapses, 76, 79–80, 276

"taking the edge off," 139
tea, 282–83
technology and Resonant, 57–58
templates (relational), Resonant,
    236–43, 245
thalamus, 58
"thought superiority" messages,
    232–33
three rules of brain change. *See* brain
    change, three rules of
tinnitus, 72–73, 74
tofu, brain's texture, 278–79
training programs, brain, 283–84
transcranial magnetic stimulation, 50
traumatized people note, 93
"trying on" a relationship, 94

If you enjoyed this book, visit

www.tarcherbooks.com

and sign up for Tarcher's e-newsletter to receive special offers, giveaway promotions, and information on hot upcoming releases.

TARCHER
PENGUIN

Great Lives Begin with Great Ideas

Connect with the Tarcher Community

• • •

Stay in touch with favorite authors!
Enter weekly contests!
Read exclusive excerpts!
Voice your opinions!

Follow us

 Tarcher Books

@TarcherBooks

If you would like to place a bulk order of this book, call 1-800-847-5515.

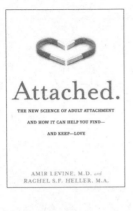

"A groundbreaking book that redefines what it means to be in a relationship."
—John Gray, Ph.D., bestselling author *of* *Men Are from Mars, Women Are from Venus*

978-1-58542-913-4

$15.95

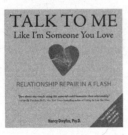

The bestselling authors of *Energy Medicine* and *Energy Medicine for Women* present a complete program for using energy medicine to heal and strengthen romantic relationships.

978-1-58542-949-3

$27.95

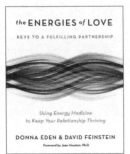

"The most crucial relationship advice book since *Men Are from Mars*."
—Erin Meanley, Glamour.com

978-0-39916-200-8

$17.95

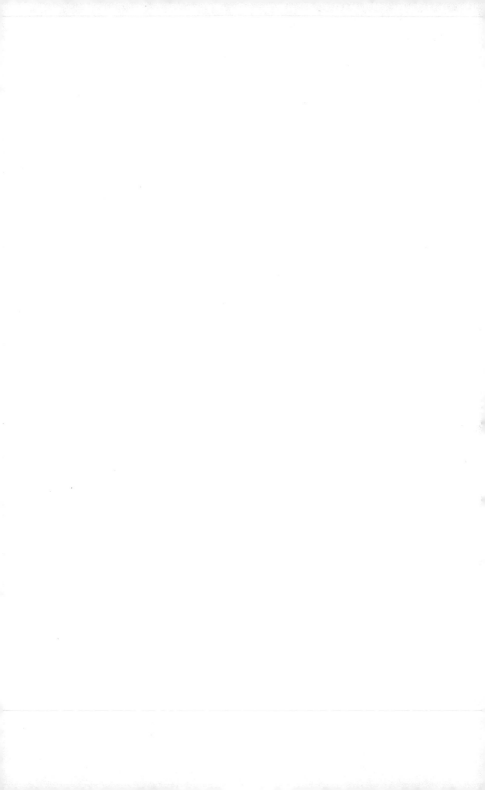